Contents

OSCEsmart

50 medical student OSCEs in Medicine

Dr Cathryn Mainwaring

BMBS (Hons.) BMedSci (Hons.) MRCP (UK)

Executive Consulting Editor:

Dr. Sam Thenabadu

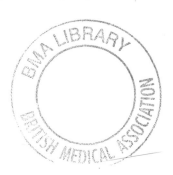
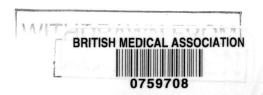

Ordering Information: Quantity sales. Special discounts are available on quantity purchases by corporations, associations, and others. For details, contact the publisher at the address above.

Orders by UK trade bookstores and wholesalers please visit
www.scowenpublishing.com

Although every effort has been made to check this text, it is possible that errors have been made, readers are urged to check with the most up to date guidelines and safety regulations.

The authors and the publishers do not accept responsibility or legal liability for any errors in the text, or for the misuse of the material in this book.

Publisher's Cataloging-in-Publication data : OSCEsmart 50 medical student OSCEs in Medicine.

ISBN-10: 0-9985267-0-3
ISBN-13: 978-0-9985267-0-6

Message from the authors

Doctors of all seniorities can remember the stress of the OSCEs but even more so the stress of trying to study and practice for the OSCE. A multitude of generic undergraduate and postgraduate resources can be found online but quality, quantity, and completeness of content can vary. The aim of the OSCESmart editorial team is to bring together specialty focused books that have identified 50 core stations encompassing the essential categories of history taking, examinations, emergency moulages, clinical skills and data interpretation with a strong theme of communications running through all the stations.

The combined experience of consultants, registrars and junior doctors to write, edit and quality check these stations, promises to deliver content that is appropriate to reach a standard we would expect of new junior doctors entering their foundation internship years and into core training. It is important to know that these stations are all newly written and based at the level of clinical competencies we would expect from these grades of doctors. Learning objectives exist for undergraduate curricula and for the foundation years, and the scenarios are based and written around these. What they are not, are scenarios that have been 'borrowed' from any medical school.

Preparation is the key to success in most things, but never more so than for the OSCEs and a candidate that hasn't practised will soon be found out. These books will allow you to practice relevant scenarios with verified checklists to learn both content and the generic approach. The format will allow you to practice in groups with one person being the candidate, one the actor and one the examiner. Each scenario finishes with three learning points. Picture these as are three core learning tips that we would want you to take away if you had only a couple of days left to the exam. These OSCE scenarios promise to be a robust revision aide for the student looking to recap and consolidate for their exams, but equally importantly prepare them for life in clinical practice.

I am immensely proud of this OSCESmart series. I have had the pleasure of working with some of the brightest and most dynamic young clinicians and educators I know, and I am sure you will find this series covering the essential clinical specialties a truly robust and invaluable companion in those stressful times of revision. I must take this opportunity to thank my colleagues for all their hard work but most of all to thank my wonderful wife Molly for her unerring love and support and my sons Reuben and Rafael for all the joy they bring me.

Despite the challenging times the health service finds itself in, being a doctor remains a huge privilege. We hope that this OSCESmart series goes some way to help you achieve the excellence you and your patients deserve.

Best of luck, Dr Sam Thenabadu

Introduction to OSCESmart 50 OSCEs: OSCES in Medicine

I remember very clearly my final year OSCE's at medical school. The mixed feelings of anticipation and dread. Wanting to get this rite of passage out of the way, but equally not wanting to let myself down at this final hurdle after months of preparation. We had established an "OSCE Group" and met regularly to practice at each other's houses. The checklists we used were ones that had been passed down through generations of medical students, or that we had devised ourselves. However, uncertainty pervaded and we had no idea what to expect. If only we had had a revision aid such as this all those years ago.

This book aims to give you a taster of the structure and approach that you should use at different types of OSCE station. It is divided into acute stations, clinical examinations, data interpretation, practical skills, history taking and communication skills sections. Covering a wide breadth of different OSCE stations that you may encounter

It is impossible to cover the whole of the medical curriculum in one book, so we have had to use common examples where appropriate. However, I hope that you will be able to use the structured approach given in the mark scheme to attempt any OSCE station or tackle any clinical problem. For example, the structured approach used to interpret a chest x-ray showing a pleural effusion, will be same as that used to interpret an x-ray showing a pneumothorax.

The strength of this book is that it has been written and researched by newly qualified foundation doctors, who hail from a variety of medical schools. Having recent experience of modern day OSCE examinations and cases, only adds to the validity of this book as a revision aid; my thanks to them for all their hard work in putting this book together.

My final thanks go to my partner Charlie and my parents for putting up with my never ending academic endeavours, to my friend and mentor Dr Sam Thenabadu for giving me this opportunity, and my old OSCE group girls (you know who you are).

Finally, I hope that you find this book a useful revision aid and myself and my team would like to wish you all the best in your forthcoming examinations, and future careers.

Cathryn

Dr Cathryn Mainwaring

BM BS (Hons.) BMedsci (Hons.) MRCP (UK)

About the authors

Dr Cathryn Mainwaring

BM BS (Hons.) BMedsci (Hons.) MRCP (UK)

Cathryn graduated from the University of Nottingham Medical School with an Honours degree in 2009. After completing her foundation training in the East Midlands she spent 9 months working in the Emergency Department of the National University Hospital Singapore. She returned to the East Midlands in 2012 to complete core medical training. In 2014 she moved to the London Deanery to take up a training number in Geriatrics.

She has an interest in medical education and is currently working as a Medical Education Fellow at King's College Hospital NHS Foundation Trust, whilst studying for a Diploma in Medical Education.

Dr Sam Thenabadu

MBBS MRCP DRCOG DCH MA Clin Ed FCEM MSc (Paed) FHEA

Consultant Adult & Paediatric Emergency Medicine
Honorary Senior Lecturer & Associate Director of Medical Education

Sam Thenabadu graduated from King's College Medical School in 2001 and dual trained in Adult and Paediatric Emergency Medicine in London before being appointed a consultant in 2011 at the Princess Royal University Hospital. He has Masters degrees in Clinical Medical Education and Advanced Paediatrics.

He is undergraduate director of medical education at the King's College NHS Trust and the academic block lead for Emergency Medicine and Critical Care at King's College School of Medicine. At postgraduate level he has been the Pan London Health Education England lead for CT3 paediatric emergency medicine trainees since 2011. Academically he has previously written two textbooks and has published in peer review journals and given numerous oral and poster presentations at national conferences in emergency medicine, paediatrics, medical education and patient quality and safety.

He has an unashamed passion for medical education and strives to achieve excellence for himself, his colleagues and his patients, hoping to always deliver this through an enjoyable learning environment. Service delivery and educational need not be two separate entities, and he hopes that those who have had great teachers will take it upon themselves to do the same for others in the future.

Abbreviations

ABG	Arterial blood gas
ABPI	Ankle-Brachial Pressure Index
AV	arteriovenous
AXR	Abdominal x-ray
BP	Blood pressure
BNP	Brain natriuretic peptide
CPR	Cardiopulmonary resuscitation
CXR	Chest x-ray
DNACPR	Do not attempt cardiopulmonary resuscitation
ECG	electrocardiogram
ESR	Erythrocyte Sedimentation Rate
FBC	Full blood count
GALS	Gait arms legs and spine
GI	Gastrointestinal
GP	General practice/ General Practicioner
G&S	Group and Save
ITU	Intensive Therapy Unit
IV	Intravenous
LFTs	Liver function tests
L/S	Lying and standing
NG	Nasogastric
NSTEMI	Non-ST-elevation myocardial infarction
PALs	Patient Advice and Liasion service
PMHx	Past medical history
STEMI	ST-elevation myocardial infarction
TFTs	Thyroid function tests
TIA	Transient ischaemic attack
T2DM	Type 2 Diabetes
U&E	Urea and Electrolytes

Co-authors' Page

Dr Rebekah Davis MBChB BMedSci, GP Specialist Trainee Year 1

Dr Samantha Fleury BMBS, Foundation Year Two Doctor

Dr Erin Kamp MBBS, Foundation Year Two Doctor

Dr Rupinder Kaur Gill MBBS, Foundation Year Two Doctor

Dr Daniella Osaghae MBBS BSc. (Hons.), Foundation Year Two Doctor

Dr Radhika Patel MBBS BSc. (Hons.), Foundation Year Two Doctor

Dr Saranya Ravindran MBBS BSc. (Hons.), Foundation Year Two Doctor

Dr Aarthi Ravishankar MBBS BSc. (Hons.), Foundation Year Two Doctor

Dr Chloe Wilkes, BMBS BMedSci, Foundation Year Two Doctor

Acute Stations

Cardiac Arrest (Shockable Rhythm)

Candidate's Instructions

You are the foundation year doctor on the cardiac arrest team. A cardiac arrest call to an adult patient on the coronary care unit has just been put out. When you arrive on the scene you find the patient unresponsive. There is a student nurse with the patient who is available to help you, but she has not commenced any treatment. The rest of the cardiac arrest team have not arrived. You are using an automated -external defibrillator.

With 1 minute remaining you will be asked to summarise to the senior team member.

Examiner's Instructions

The foundation year doctor has been called to a cardiac arrest on the coronary care unit. There is a student nurse present to assist the doctor but they have not commenced any treatment.

When the candidate attaches the AED the patient is in a shockable rhythm. The candidate is using an automated external defibrillator and is expected to perform at the level of an individual who has completed Basic Life Support Training. After delivering a shock the patient begins to show signs of life.

You may need to advance the candidate on to the next step so that they can demonstrate all the skills required.

At 7 minutes ask the patient to hand-over to you as a senior member of the cardiac arrest team.

Actor's Instructions

You are the student nurse looking after this patient. You know that he has been admitted 30 minutes ago with an acute ST-elevation myocardial infarction (STEMI) and has already received morphine, aspirin and GTN with good response. He was being prepared for the cath-lab when he complained of feeling unwell and became unresponsive.

You are able to help the junior doctor with tasks if they ask for help.

After the junior doctor administers a shock you notice that the patient is groaning and showing signs of life.

Cardiac Arrest (Shockable Rhythm)

Task	Achieved	Not Achieved
Ensures personal safety (apron and gloves)		
Checks for patient response		
Opens the airway (head tilt, chin lift)		
Calls for help		
Starts chest compressions		
Chest compressions of adequate rate 100-120/min		
Chest compressions of adequate depth 5-6cm		
Gives 30 chest compressions		
Gives 2 rescue breaths (may use barrier device)		
Does not take more than 10 seconds to deliver rescue breaths		
Recommences chest compressions		
Continues CPR at a ratio of 30:2		
Once AED arrives attaches defibrillation pads with minimal delay to compressions		
Follows AED instructions for rhythm check (shock advised)		
Performs appropriate safety checks		
Delivers safe shock		
Recommences CPR Immediately		
Discontinues CPR when patient shows signs of life		
Commences ABCDE assessment		
Safe handover to cardiac arrest team		
Examiner's Global Mark	/5	
Actor's Global Mark	/5	
Total station Mark	/30	

Learning Points

- Good quality chest compressions are the most important feature of effective cardiopulmonary resuscitation. Ensure your chest compressions are of an adequate rate and depth, and that you minimise the amount of time off the chest.

- It is important that you know how to deliver a safe shock, ensuring that oxygen has been removed and that nobody is contact with the patient or the bed. Without causing a time delay ensure you have checked at the top, middle and bottom of the patient before delivering your shock.

- Good team working is essential to a resuscitation attempt. Ensure you use clear specific instructions and communicate well with your helper or team. Closed loop communication of asking for a task to be done, checking they acknowledged and understood the task and finally ensuring that they feed back when the task is completed is the essence of good communication.

Anaphylaxis

Candidate's Instructions

You are the foundation year doctor on call for medicine. You have been called urgently to the acute medical unit to assess a patient who has suddenly become short of breath, wheezy and developed a rash.

With 2 minutes remaining the examiner will stop you and ask you to summarise your findings and ask you some direct questions.

Examiner's Instructions

The candidate is a foundation doctor who has been urgently called to the acute medical unit to assess an unwell patient. The patient has a penicillin allergy and has just been commenced on an intravenous flucloxacillin infusion to treat a case of severe cellulitis. The nurse was extremely busy and did not run through their standard allergy checks before administering the antibiotic.

Shortly after starting the infusion the patient started to complain of feeling unwell. They have developed swelling of the lips and tongue, an urticarial rash, respiratory distress and wheeze.

The candidate should recognise that this is anaphylaxis, and start emergency management as appropriate.

If the candidate asks for observations please supply them with the following information:

	Pre-treatment	Delayed Treatment	Post- Treatment (adrenaline, oxygen, fluids)
Saturations	90% on air	88% on air	98% on 15L NRB
Respiratory Rate	24	28	22
Heart Rate	120	140	130
Blood Pressure	85/40	75/32	100/80
Capillary Refill Time	4 seconds	4 seconds	3 seconds
Temperature	37.4	37.4	37.4
Blood Sugar	5.6	5.6	5.6

You may act as a second pair of hands to assist the candidate if they call for help.
At 6 minutes stop the candidate and ask how they would like to further manage the patient.

Actor's Instructions

You have been admitted with cellulitis that requires treatment with intravenous antibiotics. You have an allergy to penicillin. You have just been commenced on an infusion of intravenous flucloxacillin and have started to feel unwell. You noticed that the nurse was busy when they started the infusion, as they did not check your red wristband or allergy status.

You feel as though your tongue and lips are swollen. You feel itchy and have noticed a bumpy rash over your chest. You are finding it difficult to breathe and your chest feels tight.

If the candidate correctly recognises anaphylaxis and administers IM adrenaline, oxygen and fluids you start to feel better and less wheezy.

Anaphylaxis

Task	Achieved	Not Achieved
Ensures personal safety (apron and gloves)		
Makes general end of the bed assessment		
Introduces self to patient		
Calls for help early		
Assesses airway		
Applies high flow oxygen (15L via a non-rebreathe mask)		
Assesses breathing (RR, Trachea, Percussion, Auscultation, sats)		
Assesses circulation (CRT, HR, BP)		
Cannulates patient		
Commences IV fluid challenge (500ml-100ml IV crystalloid)		
Assesses disability (Pupils, AVPU, Blood Sugar)		
Exposes patient (identifies rash, and antibiotic infusion)		
Stops antibiotic infusion		
Gives 500 micrograms of 1:1000 Adrenaline IM		
Reassesses patient using ABCDE approach		
Gives 200mg IV Hydrocortisone		
Gives 10mg IV Chlorphenamine		
Contacts senior (medical registrar, intensive care registrar)		
Maintains communication with patient throughout		
Able to discuss further management of patient (monitoring, steroids, change of antibiotics, incident report form, duty of candour etc.)		
Examiner's Global Mark	/5	
Actor's Global Mark	/5	
Total station Mark	/30	

Learning Points

- Remember to stick to an ABCDE approach to assessment in your acute/ emergency OSCE stations. A systematic approach will prevent you from missing clinical points. After any intervention do remember to reassess the impact of your intervention.

- Apply high flow oxygen and call for help early for any sick patient. Time flies in real life (and the OSCE) so putting out a call once you have ascertained the level of severity is essential.

- The 1st line treatment of anaphylaxis includes imtra muscular (not intravenous) adrenaline, fluids and high flow oxygen. A second dose of IM adrenaline can be given after 5 minutes if there is an ongoing reaction. 2nd Line treatment includes hydrocortisone and chlorphenamine.

Sepsis

Candidate's Instructions

You are the foundation year doctor on the admitting medical team. You have been asked to assess a gentleman in the emergency department that the triage nurse is concerned about. The patient is an elderly gentleman who has been admitted generally unwell, confused and pyrexial. The district nurse changed his long-term catheter yesterday. His family say that he was well yesterday and the confusion is new.

With 2 minutes remaining the examiner will stop you and ask you to summarise your findings and ask you some direct questions.

Examiner's Instructions

The candidate is a foundation year doctor who has been asked to assess an unwell patient in the emergency department. The patient has been admitted with a short history of confusion, fever and is generally unwell. The nurse in triage has asked the candidate to assess the patient, as she is concerned.

The candidate should recognise that this patient could have sepsis, and start emergency management as appropriate.

If the candidate asks for observations please supply them with the following information:

	Pre-treatment	Delayed Treatment	Post- Treatment (oxygen, fluids, antibiotics)
Saturations	95% on air	94% on air	98% on 15L via NRB
Respiratory Rate	26	30	24
Heart Rate	115	125	101
Blood Pressure	90/65	72/55	103/70
Capillary Refill Time	4 seconds	5 seconds	3 seconds
Temperature	38.5	38.6	37.9
Blood Sugar	8.4	8.4	8.4

You may act as a second pair of hands to assist the candidate if they call for help.

When the candidate cannulates and takes bloods, please prompt to ask which bloods they would take if needed.

If the candidate requests a catheter set, or attempts to perform the procedure, please move them on.

At 6 minutes stop the candidate and ask how they would like to further manage the patient in particular the "Sepsis 6".

Actor's Instructions

You have been bought the emergency department by your family who are concerned. You have been feeling generally unwell since yesterday after the district nurse changed your long-term catheter. You are shaky, feverish and not your normal self. You are disorientated to time and place but are not known to have any memory problems.

If the candidate correctly recognises that you have sepsis and administers oxygen, IV fluids and antibiotics you start to feel better.

Sepsis

Task	Achieved	Not Achieved
Ensures personal safety (apron and gloves)		
Makes general end of the bed assessment		
Introduces self to patient		
Calls for help		
Assesses airway		
Applies high flow oxygen (15L via a NRB Mask)		
Assesses breathing (RR, Trachea, Percussion, Auscultation, Saturations)		
Assesses circulation (CRT, HR, BP)		
Cannulates patient		
Takes bloods including lactate		
Takes blood cultures		
Commences IV fluid challenge (500ml-100ml IV crystalloid)		
Assesses disability (Pupils, AVPU, Blood Sugar)		
Requests temperature		
Exposes patient		
Commences appropriate broad-spectrum IV antibiotics		
Catheterises patient and monitors urine output		
Reassesses patient using ABCDE approach		
Able to list "Sepsis 6" Components		
Able to describe further management including close monitoring, ongoing IV antibiotics and ITU review if BP not responding to fluid resuscitation.		
Examiner's Global Mark	/5	
Actor's Global Mark	/5	
Total station Mark	/30	

Learning Points

- Sepsis is a common presentation to both primary and secondary care. Sepsis management has evolved and early warning scores play a key part in knowing when and how to intervene. Red flag and Amber flag sepsis are two recent terms that have been validated. Red flag features include: Reduced conscious level to voice or pain only, new confusion, Systolic BP <90, HR >130, RR >25, Oxygen to keep saturations >92%, a non blanching rash, Anuria for >18 hours or recent chemotherapy.

- The management of sepsis must be done efficiently. An easy way to do this is to think of the sepsis 6 as "3 in and 3 out";

IN	OUT
Oxygen	Blood Cultures
Fluids	Lactate
Antibiotics	Urine Output

- Patients with a serum lactate >4mmol/L should be referred to critical care. As a junior doctor it is important to know the early pointers to stratifying how ill a patient is. Early escalation to seniors and specialists can reduce patient morbidity and mortality.

GI Bleed

Candidate's Instructions

You are the foundation year doctor on the liver ward. You have been called urgently to assess a patient who is having haematemesis and melena. The nurse tells you that the patient is known to have cirrhosis with portal hypertension and varices.

With 2 minutes remaining the examiner will stop you and ask you to summarise your findings and ask you some direct questions.

Examiner's Instructions

The candidate is a foundation doctor who has been asked to assess a patient with haematemesis and melena on the liver ward. The patient is known to have cirrhosis with portal hypertension and varices. The patient has signs of chronic liver disease and evidence of haematemesis and melena on examination.

The candidate should recognise that this patient is having an upper GI bleed (most likely variceal in origin) and start appropriate emergency management.

If the candidate asks for observations please supply them with the following information:

	Pre-treatment	Delayed Treatment	Post-Treatment (antibiotics, fluid, blood)
Saturations	94% on air	94% on air	98% on 15L NRB
Respiratory Rate	25	25	24
Heart Rate	120	125	110
Blood Pressure	81/69	73/62	90/70
Capillary Refill Time	4 seconds	5 seconds	3 seconds
Temperature	36.5	36.5	36.5
Blood Sugar	6.2	6.2	6.2

You may act as a second pair of hands to assist the candidate if they call for help.

When the candidate cannulates and takes bloods, please prompt to ask which bloods they would take if needed.

If the candidate requests the results of a venous blood gas please tell them that the haemoglobin is 65g/L

If the candidate requests a catheter set, or attempts to perform the procedure, please move them on.

At 6 minutes stop the candidate and ask how they would like to further manage the patient.

Actor's Instructions

You are known to have scarring of the liver and have had bleeding from your gullet before that they have fixed with a camera and some "elastic bands". You started vomiting a large amount of fresh red blood today, and are passing thick, black tarry stools that smell. You are feeling unwell and dizzy. You do not have any abdominal pain.

On examination you are tachypnoeic and have blood around your mouth. You have generalised abdominal tenderness, but no guarding or peritonism. You have been incontinent and there is melena in the bed. You have bilateral palmar erythema, spider naevi over your upper chest and are jaundice.

GI Bleed

Task	Achieved	Not Achieved
Ensures personal safety (apron and gloves)		
Makes general end of the bed assessment		
Introduces self to patient		
Calls for Help		
Assesses airway		
Applies high flow oxygen (15L via a non-rebreathe mask)		
Assesses breathing (RR, Trachea, Percussion, Auscultation, Saturations)		
Assesses circulation (CRT, HR, BP)		
Cannulates patient using a large bore cannula		
Takes bloods including FBC, UE, LFTs, Clotting, Lactate, Group and Save)		
Requests 2nd large bore cannula		
Commences IV fluid challenge (500ml-100ml IV crystalloid)		
Assesses disability (Pupils, AVPU, Blood Sugar)		
Exposes patient		
Requests emergency blood/ activates Major haemorrhage transfusion protocol		
Reassesses patient using ABCDE approach		
Considers the use of broad spectrum antibiotics		
Considers the use of IV terlipressin		
Contacts the emergency endoscopist on-call		
Able to describe further management including close monitoring, transfusion, ITU review and endoscopy		
Examiner's Global Mark	/5	
Actor's Global Mark	/5	
Total station Mark	/30	

Learning Points

- Have a high index of suspicion for a variceal bleed in patients with a history of liver disease and clinical signs of chronic liver disease.

- "Replace like with like" and "switch off the tap". In the actively bleeding patient fluid resuscitation is a temporary measure; ultimately they will need blood. Endoscopy is required to identify a source of bleeding and provide definitive haemostasis.

- In contrast to other patients with an upper GI Bleed, patients with known or suspected varices require the administration of prophylactic broad-spectrum antibiotics and terlipressin (a splanchnic vasoconstrictor that reduces portal hypertension).

Asthma

Candidate's Instructions

You are the foundation year doctor on respiratory ward. You have been called urgently by the nurse. She would like you to assess a 25-year-old female asthmatic that has been admitted directly to the ward. The patient has not yet received any treatment. The nurse is concerned as she is very breathless.

Please assess the patient and commence management as appropriate.

With 2 minutes remaining the examiner will stop you and ask you to summarise your findings and ask you some direct questions.

Examiner's Instructions

The candidate is a foundation year doctor who has been urgently called to the respiratory ward to assess an unwell patient. The patient is a 25-year-old female brittle asthmatic. She has been admitted directly to the ward and has not yet received any treatment. She has features of a severe asthma exacerbation.

The candidate should recognise that this is a severe exacerbation of asthma, and start emergency management as appropriate.

If the candidate asks for observations please supply them with the following information:

	Pre-treatment	Delayed Treatment	Post- Treatment (adrenaline, oxygen, fluids)
Saturations	94% on air	92% on air	98% on 15L NRB
Respiratory Rate	28	32	22
Heart Rate	115	120	115
Blood Pressure	110/70	100/85	115/70
Capillary Refill Time	2 seconds	2 seconds	2 seconds
Temperature	37.2	37.2	37.2
Blood Sugar	5.0	5.0	5.0
PEFR	180L/min	110L/min	200L/min

If the candidate performs an ABG please give them these results

pH	**7.607**		[	7.350	-	7.450	]
pCO_2	**3.00**	kPa	[	4.00	-	6.50	]
pO_2	**8.4**	kPa	[	12.0	-	15.0	]
Acid Base Status							
HCO_3^-	**22**	mmol/L	[	22	-	28	]
BE	**-6.1**	mmol/L	[	-3.0	-	3.0	]
Oximetry Values							
Hb	**135**	g/L	[	135	-	175	]
SaO_2	**94.0**	%	[	95.0	-	100.0	]
Electrolyte Values							
K^+	**4.2**	mmol/L	[	3.5	-	5.0	]
Na^+	**140**	mmol/L	[	135	-	145	]
ion Ca^{2+}	**1.15**	mmol/L	[	1.10	-	1.35	]
Cl^-	**102**	mmol/L	[	96	-	106	]
Anion Gap	**16.0**	mmol/L	[	8.0	-	16.0	]
Metabolic Values							
Lact	**1.0**	mmol/L	[	0.5	-	2.0	]
Bili	**6**	µmol/L	[		-		]

You may act as a second pair of hands to assist the candidate if they call for help. At 6 minutes stop the candidate and ask how they would like to further manage the patient.

Actor's Instructions

You have just been admitted to the respiratory ward with an exacerbation of asthma. You are known to have brittle asthma and have had several hospital admissions requiring nebulisers and steroids already this year. You have been admitted to intensive care twice before but have managed to avoid intubation and ventilation so far. You do not have any other medical problems and you do not have any allergies to any medications. You normally take a brown inhaler twice a day and a blue one as needed. You are also taking tablets for your asthma called Montelukast (leukotriene receptor antagonist) and Phyllocontin (contains theophylline). At your best your peak flow is 400L/min.

You have been feeling increasingly short of breath and wheezy for the past 2 days. It all started with a runny nose and cough, but has quickly spread to your chest. You have increased the use of your blue inhaler at home, but without any relief.

When you are examined you are breathless, and unable to complete your answers to their questions in full sentences. You are working hard but holding your own at present. There is no tracheal deviation and there is bilateral wheeze on the chest. You do not have any chest pain.

If the candidate correctly recognises asthma and commences oxygen, nebulised bronchodilators and steroids you start to feel better and but remain very wheezy and breathless.

Asthma

Task	Achieved	Not Achieved
Ensures personal safety (apron and gloves)		
Makes general end of the bed assessment		
Introduces self to patient		
Calls for help		
Assesses airway		
Applies high flow oxygen (15L via a non-rebreathe mask)		
Checks tracheal position		
Assesses breathing (RR, Percussion, Auscultation, sats)		
Measures peak flow		
Requests 5mg salbutamol, nebulised through oxygen		
Requests 500 micrograms ipratropium, nebulised through oxygen		
Assesses circulation (CRT, HR, BP)		
Assesses disability (Pupils, AVPU, Blood Sugar)		
Exposes patient		
Requests 40mg oral prednisolone or 100mg IV hydrocortisone		
Reassesses the patient using an ABCDE approach		
Requests further salbutamol nebuliser		
Escalates for senior Advice		
Considers the use of Magnesium Sulphate 2g		
Able to discuss further management of patient (monitoring, steroids, regular nebulisers, intensive care review)		
Examiner's Global Mark	/5	
Actor's Global Mark	/5	
Total station Mark	/30	

Learning Points

- The British Thoracic Society provides guidelines on how to stratify and manage acute asthma. Revise the features of an acute severe and life threatening exacerbation of asthma.

- CXR are not routinely recommended in the assessment of an asthma patient unless there is a suspected pneumothorax, consolidation, life threatening features or need for intubation and ventilation.

- IV hydrocortisone may be given if the patient is too breathless to swallow, but there is no difference in onset of action between this and oral prednisolone.

Clinical Examinations

Respiratory Examination

Candidate's Instructions

You are the foundation year doctor in respiratory clinic. Your consultant has asked you to examine a patient and report back your findings. Jim is a 75-year-old gentleman who worked in a shipyard his whole life before retiring 15 years ago. He has noticed that he has become increasingly short of breath on exertion and has a dry tickly cough.

With 2 minutes remaining the examiner will stop you and ask you to summarise your findings and ask you some direct questions.

Examiner's Instructions

The candidate has been asked to examine the patient and report back their findings. The patient has a history of occupational asbestos exposure and a history suggestive of pulmonary fibrosis. When the candidate examines the patient they find clubbing, reduced chest expansion and bilateral basal fine crackles, which do not change in character on coughing.

At 6 minutes please stop the candidate and ask them to present their findings.

Actor's Instructions

You are Jim a 75-year-old gentleman. You have been referred to the respiratory clinic as you have been experiencing increasing breathlessness on exertion and a dry tickly cough, over many months. You worked in a shipyard building ships from the age of 16 until 15 years ago when you retired.

You are not in any pain, and are happy to be examined.

Mark Scheme

Task	Achieved	Not Achieved
Washes Hands		
Introduces themselves and clarifies the patient's details		
Gains consent to examine		
Asks the patient if they have any pain		
Exposes and positions the patient		
Inspects the patient and surrounding area from the end of the bed		
Examines hands and check for the presence of asterixis		
Checks pulse		
Counts respiratory rate		
Inspects the eyes and mouth		
Examines for cervical lymph nodes		
Palpates for tracheal position		
Inspects the chest wall		
Assesses chest expansion		
Performs percussion		
Auscultates		
Performs vocal resonance		
Examines for peripheral oedema		
Thanks the patient		
Presents findings		
Examiner's global mark	/5	
Actor's global mark	/5	
Total station mark	/30	

Learning Points

- Stick to the structure; inspection, palpation, percussion, auscultation

- Remember to inspect, palpate, percuss and auscultate the anterior and posterior chest wall including the apices.

- Clubbing in a respiratory patient may be caused by lung cancer, pulmonary fibrosis or chronic suppurative lung disease (empyema, cystic fibrosis, bronchiectasis)

Cardiovascular Examination

Candidate's Instructions

You are the foundation year doctor in cardiology clinic. Your consultant has asked you to examine a patient and report back your findings. Mable is a 80-year-old female who has come for her annual check up. Her past medical history includes rheumatic fever as a child.

With 2 minutes remaining the examiner will stop you and ask you to summarise your findings and ask you some direct questions.

Examiner's Instructions

The candidate has been asked to examine the patient and report back their findings. The patient has a history of rheumatic fever as a child and has attended for a check up. When the candidate examines the patient they find an irregularly irregular pulse at a rate of 85, a displaced apex beat, a pan-systolic murmur heard loudest in the mitral area that radiates into the axilla. There are no features of heart failure.

If the candidate requests the blood pressure please tell them that it is 135/70mmHg

At 6 minutes please stop the candidate and ask them to present their findings.

Actor's Instructions

You are Mable an 80 year-old-female. You have attended the cardiology clinic for your yearly check up. You have a history of rheumatic fever as a child. You have been feeling well in yourself.

You have an irregularly irregular pulse at a rate of 85 bpm. You have a displaced apex beat and a pan-systolic murmur that is heard loudest in the mitral area and radiates into the axilla. You do not have any features suggestive of heart failure.

You are not in any pain, and are happy to be examined.

Mark Scheme

Task	Achieved	Not Achieved
Washes Hands		
Introduces themselves and clarifies the patient's details		
Gains consent to examine		
Asks the patient if they have any pain		
Exposes and positions the patient		
Inspects the patient and surrounding area from the end of the bed		
Examines hands		
Checks the radial pulse commenting on rate, rhythm, character		
Checks for a collapsing pulse		
Requests the blood pressure		
Inspects the face, eyes and mouth		
Assesses the JVP (and checks for hepatojugular reflux)		
Inspects the precordium		
Palpates apex beat		
Palpates for parasternal heave and thrills		
Auscultates in the aortic, pulmonary, tricuspid and mitral areas		
Auscultates the lung bases		
Examines for sacral and peripheral oedema		
Thanks the patient		
Presents findings		
Examiner's global mark	/5	
Actor's global mark	/5	
Total station mark	/30	

Learning Points

- If you identify a murmur it is important to comment on the timing (systolic or diastolic), location and radiation.

- The location of the apex beat may help you to differentiate between aortic stenosis and mitral regurgitation. In aortic stenosis the apex beat stays put. In mitral regurgitation the apex beat relocates.

- The murmur of mitral regurgitation radiates into the axilla. The murmur of aortic stenosis radiates to the carotids. Utilising these clues can help you differentiate the murmurs with greater confidence.

Abdominal Examination

Candidate's Instructions

You are the foundation year doctor in renal clinic. Sarah is a 42-year-old female with type 1-diabetes who has attended for review.

Your consultant has asked you to examine Sarah and report back your findings.

With 2 minutes remaining the examiner will stop you and ask you to summarise your findings and ask you some direct questions.

Examiner's Instructions

The candidate has been asked to examine the patient and report back their findings. The patient has a history of a renal transplantation for end stage renal failure caused by diabetes. She has previously had haemodialysis via a left sided radio-cephalic fistula that is no longer in use.

When the candidate examines the patient they find finger pricks in keeping with blood glucose testing, a left radio-cephalic fistula with no evidence of recent use, a hockey-shaped scar in the right iliac fossa and a with an underlying palpable mass that is non-tender.

At 6 minutes please stop the candidate and ask them to present their findings.

Actor's Instructions

You are Sarah a 42-year-old female. You have a history of type 1 diabetes and end-stage renal failure. You have previously had haemodialysis via a radiocephalic fistula on your left arm. The fistula is still functioning but is not longer in use, and there are no evident needling marks or "button holes". You have had a successful renal transplantation. Your graft is located in the right iliac fossa and is non-tender.

You are not in any pain, and are happy to be examined.

Mark Scheme

Task	Achieved	Not Achieved
Washes Hands		
Introduces themselves and clarifies the patient's details		
Gains consent to examine		
Asks the patient if they have any pain		
Exposes and positions the patient		
Inspects the patient and surrounding area from the end of the bed		
Examines hands and check for the presence of asterixis		
Checks the heart rate		
Inspects the eyes and mouth		
Inspects the abdomen		
Palpates all 4 quadrants of the abdomen (superficial and deep)		
Palpates the liver		
Percusses the liver		
Palpates the spleen		
Percusses the spleen		
Ballots the kidneys bilaterally		
Palpates the "mass" (renal transplant)		
Auscultates		
Thanks the patient		
Presents findings		
Examiner's global mark	/5	
Actor's global mark	/5	
Total station mark	/30	

Learning Points

- Remember to lay the patient flat, and kneel whilst examining the abdomen. It is important to look at the patient's face whilst palpating to look for any signs of discomfort or pain.

- Tenderness over a renal transplant graft may suggest that the graft is being rejected.

- If the patient has a renal transplant look for evidence of previous renal replacement therapy (haemodialysis access or peritoneal dialysis access) and evidence of causes of end-stage renal failure such as diabetes or systemic lupus erythematosus (SLE).

Neurology Examination - Upper Limb

Candidate's Instructions

You are the foundation year doctor in the stroke outpatient clinic. John is a 72-year-old gentleman who has presented for review following a recent admission.

Your consultant has asked you to examine John and report back your findings.

With 2 minutes remaining the examiner will stop you and ask you to summarise your findings and ask you some direct questions.

Examiner's Instructions

The candidate has been asked to examine the patient and report back their findings. The patient is a 72-year-old gentleman who has been a recent inpatient on the stroke unit. He has a history of a left hemispheric ischaemic infarct that caused right-sided face, arm and leg weakness.

When the candidate examines the patient they find a right sided facial droop, a pronator drift, increased tone, reduced power (4/5) and brisk reflexes on the right hand side. Co-ordination on the right is impaired due to weakness. Sensation is intact.

At 6 minutes please stop the candidate and ask them to present their findings.

Actor's Instructions

You are John, a 72-year-old gentleman who has attended the stroke clinic for review following an admission on the stroke unit. You had a left hemispheric ischaemic infarct that caused right-sided face, arm and leg weakness. You have made a good recovery but now need to use a quad stick to walk. Your right side has improved but is still weak in comparison to your left side.

When you are examined your right arm turns over when both arms are held in the air, palms up, with your eyes closed. The right arm is stiff. It is weak in-comparison to the left side. You are able to perform tasks against gravity and resistance, but it is not as strong as the left. The reflexes in the right arm are brisk. When asked to perform coordination tasks you are able to do so accurately but you are slow and purposeful. The sensation in your arm is normal.

You are not in any pain, and are happy to be examined.

Mark Scheme

Task	Achieved	Not Achieved
Washes Hands		
Introduces themselves and clarifies the patient's details		
Gains consent to examine		
Asks the patient if they have any pain		
Exposes and positions the patient		
Inspects the patient and surrounding area from the end of the bed		
Assesses for pronator drift		
Examines tone		
Assesses power of shoulder abduction/ adduction		
Assesses power of elbow flexion/ extension		
Assesses power of wrist flexion/ extension		
Assesses power of finger abduction/ adduction		
Assesses power Grip		
Assesses biceps Reflex		
Assesses triceps Reflex		
Assesses supinator Reflex		
Tests sensation in all dermatomes		
Tests coordination		
Thanks the patient		
Presents findings		
Examiner's global mark	/5	
Actor's global mark	/5	
Total station mark	/30	

Learning Points

- Testing for pronator drift early in your examination may be an important clue to help you focus your examination.

- To remember the order of the neurology examination remember "**I**n the **P**ouring **R**ain **S**he **C**ame"; **I**nspection, **P**ower, **R**eflexes, **S**ensation, **C**oordination.

- Eliciting reflexes can be a difficult technique. Practice using the tendon hammer. Don't forget to use reinforcement before declaring that a reflex is absent.

Neurology Examination - Lower Limb

Candidate's Instructions

You are the foundation year doctor in endocrinology outpatient clinic. The next patient is a 62-year-old gentleman called Ronald.

Your consultant has asked you to examine Ronald and report back your findings.

With 2 minutes remaining the examiner will stop you and ask you to summarise your findings and ask you some direct questions.

Examiner's Instructions

Ronald is a patient with poorly controlled type 2 diabetes. He has attended the endocrinology outpatient clinic for review.

The candidate has been asked to perform a neurological examination of the lower limb and report back their findings. When the candidate examines the patient they find tone, power and coordination are normal. The ankle reflexes are absent. The patient has lost sensation bilaterally in a stocking distribution to pain, temperature and vibration. Proprioception is impaired at the great toe, but intact at the ankle. Romberg's sign is positive.

At 6 minutes please stop the candidate and ask them to present their findings.

Actor's Instructions

You are a 62-year-old gentleman called Ronald. You are a type 2 diabetic and have been since you were 51 years old. You have problems controlling your diabetes because your shift pattern as a lorry driver makes it difficult to stick to a healthy diet and take your medications regularly. Over the past year you have noticed that you have tingling burning pains in your feet, particularly at night. You have not attended your diabetic foot check because you have been too busy.

When the candidate examines you the tone and power in your lower limbs is normal. You have absent ankle reflexes. Co-ordination is normal. You have lost the sensations of light touch, pain and temperature to your mid shins in a stocking-like distribution. You have lost proprioception in your big toes bilaterally, but not in your ankle joints. You do not have any skin breaks or ulcers.

If the candidate performs a Romberg's test this is positive i.e. you start to sway and feel unsteady when asked to stand with your eyes closed and feet shoulder width apart.

Mark Scheme

Task	Achieved	Not Achieved
Washes Hands		
Introduces themselves and clarifies the patient's details		
Gains consent to examine		
Asks the patient if they have any pain		
Exposes and positions the patient		
Inspects the patient and surrounding area from the end of the bed		
Examines tone and assesses for clonus bilaterally		
Assesses power of hip flexion/ extension		
Assesses power of knee flexion/ extension		
Assesses power of dorsiflexion/ plantarflexion		
Assesses knee jerk reflexes		
Assesses ankle jerk reflexes		
Tests Babinski's sign bilaterally		
Assesses coordination		
Assesses light touch sensation		
Assesses pain and vibration sense		
Assesses proprioception		
Assesses gait and performs Romberg's test		
Thanks the patient		
Presents findings		
Examiner's global mark	/5	
Actor's global mark	/5	
Total station mark	/30	

Learning Points

- Clonus is a series of involuntary muscular contractions and relaxations. It is associated with upper motor neurone lesions and spasticity. More than 5 beats of clonus at the ankle joint are considered pathological.

- You can assess for temperature sensation using a cold object such as the metal surface of a tuning fork. When assessing vibration sense you must use a 128 Hz tuning fork.

- In diabetes (type 1 or type 2), symptoms of peripheral neuropathy are mostly sensory, with light touch, pain, temperature and proprioception the first to be affected in a glove and stocking distribution.

Cerebellar Examination

Candidate's Instructions

A 45-year-old lady comes into the emergency department with a 3 day history of worsening balance and falls. You see from her previous clinic letters that she was diagnosed with multiple sclerosis 10 years ago.

Your consultant has asked you to do a thorough cerebellar examination and present your findings.

With 2 minutes remaining the examiner will stop you and ask you to summarise your findings and ask you some direct questions.

Examiner's instructions

A 45-year-old lady comes into the emergency department with a 3 day history of poor balance and falls. She was diagnosed with multiple sclerosis 10 years ago. The foundation doctor has been asked to perform a thorough cerebellar examination and present their findings to you.

The patient has an ataxic gait, particularly on heel toe walking. Romberg's test however is negative. There is no truncal ataxia. She also has nystagmus on bilateral lateral gaze and an intention tremor on both sides. Her speech also sounds dysarthric.

At 6 minutes ask the candidate to present their findings.

Actor's instructions

You are a 45-year-old female who was diagnosed with multiple sclerosis 10 years ago. You have come to the emergency department as you feel like you have lost all sense of balance and have had several falls over the past 3 days.

On examination you have an unsteady (ataxic) gait, particularly on heel-toe walking. Romberg's Test is negative. You have a bilateral intention tremor and nystagmus on lateral gaze. Your speech also sounds slurred.

Mark Scheme

Task	Achieved	Not Achieved
Washes Hands		
Introduces themselves and clarifies the patient's details		
Gains consent to examine		
Asks the patient if they have any pain		
Exposes and positions the patient		
Inspects the patient and surrounding area from the end of the bed		
Assesses eye movements and comments on the presence/absence of nystagmus		
Assesses speech for dysarthria		
Assesses for pronator drift		
Assesses for rebound phenomenon		
Assesses tone in the upper limb		
Assesses tone in the lower limb		
Assesses coordination in the lower limb		
Assesses for truncal ataxia		
Assesses coordination in the lower limb		
Performs Romberg's Test		
Observes the patient's gait		
Asks the patient to heel-toe walk		
Thanks the patient		
Presents findings		
Examiner's Global Mark	/5	
Actor/ Helper's Global Mark	/5	
Total station mark Mark	/30	

Learning Points

- Romberg's test can help to differentiate between a cerebellar and a sensory ataxia. With a sensory ataxia the patient will become unsteady whilst standing with their eyes closed. With a cerebellar ataxia the patient will remain relatively steady whilst standing with their eyes closed.

- Truncal ataxia can be tested by asking the patient to sit on the edge of the examination couch with their arms crossed across their chest.

- If in doubt remember "DANISH"
  Dysdiadokokinesis

  Ataxia

  Nystagmus

  Intention tremor

  Slurred/ Staccato speech

  Hypotonia/ Heel-shin test

Focused Tremor Examination

Candidate's Instructions

You are the foundation year doctor in a General Practice surgery. A 78-year-old gentleman has presented with a tremor in his hands. Your trainer has asked you to examine the patient and present your findings.

With 2 minutes remaining the examiner will stop you and ask you to summarise your findings and ask you some direct questions.

Examiner's Instructions

A 78-year-old gentleman has presented to his GP with a tremor in his hands and the candidate has been asked to examine the patient.

If the candidate goes to examine the lower limbs please move them on and inform them that they only need to examine upper limbs.

If candidate asks the patient to write a sentence please ask them to move on, and give them the relevant mark.

Positive finds are:

- Resting Pill-rolling tremor worse on distraction
- Increased tone (lead pipe rigidity)
- Cogwheel rigidity
- Bradykinesia
- Shuffling gait
- Reduced arm swing
- Stooped posture
- Difficulty initiating movement
- Hypophonia (quiet voice)

At 6 minutes please stop the candidate and ask them to present their findings.

Actor's Instructions

You are a 78-year-old gentleman who has presented to his GP with a tremor. The tremor started in your right hand several years ago, but it has now spread to affect the left side.

The junior doctor has been asked to examine you, please be cooperative. You have a walking stick with you. You are not in any pain. You have a quiet, monotonous voice.

ARMS: When the candidate moves your arms around you are very stiff, with increased tone and cog-wheeling. The power in your arms is good, but every movement takes you a long time. You have difficulty with functional tasks and struggle to undo/do a button due to your tremor.

HANDS: At rest you have a 'pill-rolling' tremor, which is worse when distracted (e.g counting). When asked to do hand movements you are very slow and they get smaller and slower each time you repeat the action.

WALKING: When asked to stand you have a stooped posture and lean forwards. You have difficulty initiating movement, walk in shuffling steps and are very slow to turn around (taking lots of small shuffling steps). You do not swing your arms when you walk.

Everything else is normal (reflexes, coordination, power)

Tremor

Task:	Achieved	Not Achieved
Washes hands		
Introduces self		
Confirms name and age of patient		
Explains examination and gets consent		
Exposes patient and asks patient to sit		
Asks about pain		
Inspects surroundings for walking aids etc.		
Examines patient from end of bed		
Inspects hands for resting tremor using distraction technique		
Assesses tone of upper limbs		
Assesses power of upper limbs		
Assesses co-ordination		
Assesses for bradykinesia		
Assesses face and eye movements		
Assesses speech		
Assesses motor function e.g. undoing a button		
Asks patient to write		
Observes gait		
Offers to test balance, complete full neurological examination, cerebellar examination, L/S BP, check drug chart, assess cognitive impairment.		
Summarises and gives at least 2 correct findings		
Examiner's Global Mark	/5	
Actor / Helper's Global Mark	/5	
Total Station Mark	/30	

Learning Points

- It is likely that your patient in the exam will have real pathology. Ensure you practice with real Parkinson's patients before the exam so you feel confident and are easily able to recognise the typical features.

- The three pathognomonic features of Parkinson's disease are; bradykinesia, resting pill-rolling tremor, increased tone (lead pipe rigidity).

Other typical positive finds are:

- Cogwheel rigidity
- Shuffling gait
- Reduced arm swing
- Stooped posture
- Difficulty initiating movement
- Hypophonia (quiet voice)
- Hypomimia (expressionless face)
- Small spidery handwriting (micrographia)

- Signs such as impaired eye movements, cerebellar signs or cognitive impairment may suggest an alternative diagnosis such as one of the "Parkinson's Plus" Syndromes.

Opthalmology

Candidate's Instructions

You are the foundation year doctor in the emergency department. A 50-year old gentleman has come in with a visual changes and a headache.

You have been asked to perform a cranial nerve examination focusing on the eyes, and present your findings. You are not required to perform fundoscopy.

With 2 minutes remaining the examiner will stop you and ask you to summarise your findings and ask you some direct questions.

Examiner's Instructions

The candidate is a foundation doctor in the emergency department seeing a 50-year old gentleman who has presented with visual changes and a headache.

The candidate has been asked to examine the patient's eyes. Please provide a Snellen chart if/when the candidate asks for it.

The candidate is not required to perform fundoscopy.

At 6 minutes please stop the candidate and ask them to present their findings.

Actor's Instructions

You are a 50-year-old-gentleman. You have noticed a change in your vision for the last two weeks. You find yourself bumping into furniture around the house and at work. This has been associated with a generalized headache over the last week that has been getting worse, despite regular paracetamol and ibuprofen. You do not have blurred vision, increased sensitivity to light, or pain in or around your eyes. Prior to this, you were well. You have decided to come to the emergency department because you are concerned that your symptoms are not improving.

On examination, visual acuity is normal. Pupils are equal and reactive to light. Visual fields reveal a bitemporal hemianopia. Eye movements are normal without nystagmus or diplopia.

Opthalmology

Task:	Achieved	Not Achieved
Washes Hands		
Introduces self		
Confirms name and age of patient		
Positions patient appropriately		
Asks about pain		
Asks about any change in vision – specify characteristics.		
Inspects eyes and surrounding area		
Asks if glasses worn		
Uses Snellen chart to test visual acuity		
Offers to check colour vision with Ishihara plates		
Checks direct and consensual pupillary reflex		
Performs swinging light test		
Checks for accommodation		
Visual fields with appropriate technique: candidate hand should be equidistant from patient and candidate, and candidate should be at same level as the patient		
Tests for visual neglect		
Checks blind spot with red hat pin		
Assesses eye movements and comments on the presence of asymmetry or nystagmus		
Asks patient to report diplopia during examination of eye movements.		
Thanks patient		
Presents findings in a concise, logical manner		
Examiner's Global Mark	/5	
Actor / Helper's Global Mark	/5	
Total Station Mark	/30	

Learning Points

- Remember it is important to ask if the patient wears glasses. If they do wear glasses test visual acuity with their glasses on.

- The swinging light test assesses for the presence of a relative afferent pupillary defect (RAPD). RAPD's are caused by damage to the afferent optic pathways i.e. damage to the retina or optic nerve. Normally the pupils should hold their degree of constriction when a light is swung from one eye to the other. However, if a RAPD is present the pupil of the affected eye will appear to get larger.

- Bitemporal hemianopia is most commonly caused by a pituitary adenoma. However, any lesion at the optic chiasm (meningioma, craniopharyngioma, anterior communicating artery aneurysm) may cause this deficit. Appropriate initial investigations would include a pituitary hormone screen, formal visual fields testing, and neuroimaging.

GALS (Gait, Arms, Legs and Spine)

Candidate's Instructions

This 40-year-old gentleman has attended his GP with a long history of backache and stiffness. He has previously attributed his symptoms to his physical job as a scaffolder.

You are the foundation doctor attached to the GP surgery and have been asked to perform a screening examination of his gait, arms, legs and spine before presenting your findings to your GP trainer.

With 2 minutes remaining the examiner will stop you and ask you to summarise your findings and ask you some direct questions.

Examiner's Instructions

This 40-year-old gentleman has attended his GP with a long history of back pain and stiffness. It is essential that the candidate asks the 3 initial screening questions, but they should not go on to take a full history, as this is an examination station. They may be reminded of this if they take over 1 minute asking the 3 initial screening questions.

The candidate has been asked to perform a screening examination of his gait, arms, legs and spine before presenting their findings back to you.

At 6 minutes please stop the candidate and ask them to present their findings.

Actor's Instructions

You are a 40-year-old scaffolder. You booked a GP appointment today as the back pain and stiffness you have been experiencing for several years has got worse.

You work as a scaffolder, and previously have attributed your back problems to your work. You can be slow to get going in the mornings, but after about an hour you start to feel better. You have found that regular swimming helps. You are otherwise well, but have had a problem with inflammation of your eye in the past, that was treated with steroid drops. You do not have any difficulty climbing the stairs, but you do struggle to bend to put your shoes and socks on in the morning.

On inspection there is some thoracic kyphosis. Your gait is normal, but you do tend to turn-en-bloc. There is no bony tenderness of the vertebrae. Schober's test is positive, and you have reduced range of movements in all parts of your spine. There are no other signs.

Mark Scheme

Task:	Achieved	Not Achieved
Introduces self and washes hands		
Asks about pain or stiffness in muscles, back or joints		
Asks about ability/ difficulty in climbing stairs		
Asks about ability/ difficulty with dressing and washing		
Asks patient to undress to undergarments and explains GALS examination		
Inspects patient while standing from front, back and side to comment on spine		
Inspects gait commenting on symmetry, smoothness and turning		
Palpates for temperature and any bony tenderness of vertebrae		
Examines for forwards flexion (modified Schober's test) and spinal rotation		
Examines for flexion, extension and lateral flexion of the neck (chin on chest, ear on shoulder) and movements of the temporomandibular joints		
Inspects arms and hands (skin including nails, muscles and joints)		
Palpates hands and arms for temperature, tenderness and swelling including MCP squeeze		
Examines for power and precision grip		
Examines for wrist flexion and extension and elbow flexion and extension		
Examines for shoulder abduction and external rotation (hands behind head)		
Inspects legs (skin including nails, muscles and joints)		
Palpates for temperature, tenderness and swelling including MTP joint squeeze and patella tap		
Examines for knee flexion and extension including crepitus		
Examines for internal and external rotation of hip		
Presents findings in a concise, logical manner.		
Examiner's Global Mark	/5	
Actor / Helper's Global Mark	/5	
Total Station Mark	/30	

Learning Points

- GALS is a screening examination and always begins with the same three direct questions. It is unlikely to provide a diagnosis but should point towards which joints require further more detailed assessment.

- The initial screening questions about pain, stiffness and activities of daily living are key and can provide excellent clues in an OSCE setting. They also provide critical information about the impact of the disease on the patient.

- Prolonged morning stiffness, pain improved on activity and restricted range of movement of the spine, are common features of Ankylosing Spondylitis.

Hand Examination

Candidate's Instructions

A 45-year-old lady has been admitted to the Acute Medical Unit with a chest infection. This morning on the ward round, she mentioned that she has had pain in her hands for a few months, but has not yet seen her GP about this.

You are the foundation doctor and have been asked to perform a hand examination then present your findings back to your team.

Examiner's Instructions

A 45-year-old lady has been admitted to the Acute Medical Unit for treatment for a chest infection. Today she has mentioned to the team that she has been having pain in her hands for the past few months. Currently, the patient is not in pain. The candidate has been asked to complete a hand examination and present their findings back to you.

The patient does not have any nail, skin changes or scars. There is visible swelling over the MCP joints, PIP joints and wrists bilaterally. Temperature is increased over the swollen joints, and they are tender to palpation. The pulses are intact. The patient is able to make the prayer signs, but is unable to fully complete the range of movement. Power and sensation are intact. The patient can perform functional tasks, but they can be painful. She has some nodules on her elbows.

During the examination, as the candidate palpates the joints, the patient grimaces in pain. If candidate notices and offers analgesia, you should acknowledge this and state, "the patient has now been given pain relief, you can continue" and allow the candidate to continue examining.

At 6 minutes please stop the candidate and ask them to present their findings. Show the candidate a picture demonstrating the hand signs of rheumatoid arthritis and ask the candidate to list the deformities present.

Actor's Instructions

You are a 45-year-old lady who has been experiencing tenderness in your hands for several months. It is limiting your ability to perform normal daily tasks. It has been getting worse, but you have not yet seen your GP about. Now you have been admitted with a chest infection so you decide to mention it to the doctors looking after you on their ward round. When you are not moving your hands, you feel very little pain - so if the candidate asks you whether you are in pain at the start of the examination, say "no".

When the candidate starts to palpate your joints, you feel pain and grimace, but don't make a noise. If the candidate does not take notice of your pain, keep grimacing throughout examination then say "ouch" when you are asked to do movements of your hands. If the candidate acknowledges your pain, the examiner will ask them to proceed as if you have been given painkillers and you should then appear settled.

You do not have any nail, skin changes or scars. You do have visible swelling over the MCP joints, PIP joints and wrists bilaterally. Temperature is increased over the swollen joints, and they are tender to palpation. Your pulses are intact. You can make the prayer signs, but are unable to fully complete the range of movement. Power and sensation are intact. You are able to perform functional tasks, but they can be painful. You have some nodules on your elbows.

Hand Examination

Task:	Achieved	Not Achieved
Washes Hands		
Introduces self and clarifies patient details		
Gains informed consent for examination		
Asks the patient if they have any pain		
Positions patient with hands resting on pillow		
Looks; inspects the hands on both sides (nail changes, skin changes, scars, muscle wasting, palmar thickening, deformities and joint swelling)		
Feels; temperature of both hands		
Feels; all joints for swelling and tenderness in a systematic manner (e.g. starting proximally at radial styloid, squeezing across MCP joints and going distally to interphalangeal joints)		
Feels; ulna and radial pulses bilaterally		
Move; asks patient to make prayer sign and reverse prayer sign.		
Move; demonstrates ulnar and radial deviation		
Move; demonstrates pronation and supination		
Checks **power** of radial, ulnar and medial nerves – finger extension, finger abduction, finger adduction, thumb abduction and adduction against resistance		
Briefly checks light touch **sensation** in distribution of radial, ulnar and median nerves		
Assesses **function** – power grip and pincer grip (e.g. hold pen, button, pick up coin)		
Checks elbows for scars, rheumatoid nodules and psoriasis		
Thanks patient		
Presents findings in a concise, logical manner.		
Correctly lists common hand features of rheumatoid arthritis		
Addresses patient's pain/attends to comfort		
Examiner's Global Mark	/5	
Actor / Helper's Global Mark	/5	
Total Station Mark	/30	

Learning Points

- Always follow the principle LOOK, FEEL and MOVE in musculoskeletal examinations.

- It is important to ask about pain, acknowledge pain and then pause to offer analgesia in any examination. Look at the patient's face whilst examining, as they may not volunteer this.

- Rheumatoid arthritis and osteoarthritis are common exam cases and it is important you are confident with distinguishing between the different features of each:

Rheumatoid Arthritis	Osteoarthritis
Onset any age	Onset in old age
Autoimmune	Degenerative
Morning stiffness	Stiffness worse at end of day
Symmetrical pattern of joints affected	Asymmetrical
Classic deformities: Boutonnières, swan neck, Z-shaped thumb	Classic deformities: Bouchard's nodes (proximal), Heberden's node (distal), squaring of CMC joint of thumb
Extra-articular features e.g. rheumatoid nodules, pleural effusions, splenomegaly, nephrotic syndrome.	No systemic features. Large and small joints affected.

AV fistula

Candidate's instructions

You are the foundation year doctor in the emergency department. A known dialysis patient attends complaining of swelling in their left arm, where they also have an AV fistula in situ. You are asked by your consultant to examine the fistula and present your findings to him. The patient's observations are currently within the normal range and they are otherwise well.

With 2 minutes remaining the examiner will stop you and ask you to summarise your findings and ask you some direct questions.

Examiner's instructions

The candidate is a foundation year doctor in the emergency department. They have been asked to examine the fistula of a known dialysis patient. The patient is attending the emergency department complaining of swelling in their left arm, where they also have an AV fistula in situ. The candidate has been asked by their consultant to examine the fistula and present their findings to him.

The patient's observations are within the normal range. He has been feeling generally unwell since yesterday. There is visible erythema and swelling overlying the fistula sight. The patient has an old radiocephalic fistula that has become thrombosed and scars in the neck where they have previously required central venous access. No other abnormalities are found on examination.

At 6 minutes please stop the candidate and ask them to present their findings.

Actor's instructions

You are a haemodialysis patient, with a brachiocephalic fistula that has been in situ for 2 years. It is used for dialysis 3 times weekly. You have noticed increased swelling in your fistula arm since yesterday, mainly around the fistula site itself and have attended the emergency department for further assessment. You have been feeling generally under the weather since yesterday.

Your fistula sight looks red and swollen; it is warm to touch. There are no swelling, skin or pulse changes in your hand. You have a previous thrombosed fistula in the left radiocephalic region, and evidence of a previous central venous access with scars in your neck.

AV Fistula

Task:	Achieved	Not Achieved
Introduces self		
Correctly identifies patient		
Washes Hands		
Asks the patient if they have any pain		
Asks the patient how long the fistula has been formed and whether it is a native fistula or graft.		
Correctly identifies fistula (radiocephalic or brachiocephalic)		
Assesses skin health (Ulceration, bleeding points, sign of infection)		
Looks for recent evidence of use (needle marks-button holes or laddering-, areas of scabbing, bandage)		
Looks for any obvious swelling to arm (e.g. aneurysms, inflow/outflow obstruction)		
Looks at the hand for evidence of ischaemia (e.g. Steal Syndrome)		
Looks for evidence of old fistulas		
Looks for other IV access points e.g. long line (subclavian, cervical, femoral)		
Palpates fistula for thrill or pulse with flat of hand distal to proximal		
Palpates draining veins in upper arm and chest to feel for thrills (may indicate stenosis)		
Assesses for outflow stenosis: when arm is lifted, fistula should flatten or collapse		
Assesses for inflow stenosis: when fistula is occluded proximal to anastomosis, a pulse rather than thrill is felt over anastomosis and fistula should increase in size.		
Looks for accessory pathways: occlude fistula proximal to anastomosis and look for collateral distended veins		
Auscultates fistula to identify bruits (should be low pitched; high pitched may indicate stenosis)		
Fells the temperature and pulses of the hand		
Presents findings in a concise, logical manner.		
Examiner's global mark	/5	
Actor/Helper's global mark	/5	
Total station mark	/30	

Learning points

- Learn to identify the location of a fistula:
    - Brachiocephalic: Scar at elbow crease
    - Radiocephalic: Scar at wrist

- Remember that just because you identify an AV fistula, does not mean it is always in use: they take 3-6 months to mature. Dressings and needle marks suggest recent use. Always look for other forms of access (peritoneal or intravenous) in a patient with an AV fistula.

- Complications that may occur with an AV fistula include infection, bleeding, aneurysms, thrombosis and venous stenosis. Steal syndrome is a rare but important complication of AV fistula formation, where the distal blood supply to the limb is threatened by preferential flow of blood through the AV fistula.

Data Interpretation

ECG

Candidate's Instructions

You are a foundation year doctor in the emergency department. A 65-year-old gentleman has been brought in with a 2 hour history of crushing central chest pain. An ECG has been done as well as routine bloods.

You have been asked to interpret the ECG and explain to the patient what you have found. Please talk through your interpretation of the ECG out loud.

At 6 minutes you will be asked how you would like to assess and manage this patient.

Examiner's instructions

A 65-year-old man has attended the emergency department with a 2 hour history of central crushing chest pain. An ECG has been done as well as routine bloods.

The candidate has been asked to interpret the ECG and explain their findings to the patient. The candidate has been asked to voice their interpretation of the ECG out loud. If they do not do this please prompt them to do so.

At 6 minutes please stop the candidate and ask them how they would like to assess and manage this patient.

The candidate should identify that this is an Acute ST Elevation MI. They would assess them using an ABCDE approach. They require oxygen, morphine, nitrates, aspirin and percutaneous coronary intervention (PCI). If the candidate is doing well you may ask them which is the most likely coronary artery to have been affected.

Actor's Instructions

You are a 65 year old gentleman. You have presented to the emergency department with a 2 hour history of central crushing chest pain. An ECG and bloods have been taken. The candidate has been asked to interpret the ECG and explain their findings to you.

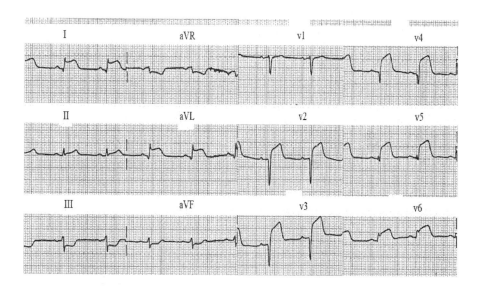

Mark Scheme

Task	Achieved	Not Achieved
Identifies patient details		
Comments of the time and date of the ECG		
Comments on the reason for the ECG e.g. "chest pain"		
Checks that the ECG is calibrated correctly (25mm/second, 10m/milli-Volt)		
Comments on the rate		
Comments on the rhythm		
Comments on the axis		
Comments on P-wave morphology		
Comments on P-R interval		
Comments on QRS duration		
Comments on ST segments		
Identifies ST elevation and which territory is affected (inferior, lateral, septal, anterior)		
Comments on T-wave morphology		
Comments on the presence/ absence of Q waves		
Makes a diagnosis of STEMI		
States initial investigations would include bedside observations, bloods including troponin and a chest x-ray		
States they would assess the patient using an ABCDE approach		
States the management would include morphine, aspirin, oxygen and nitrates		
States the patient requires urgent PCI		
Able to identify the most-likely culprit vessel		
Examiner's global mark	/5	
Actor's global mark	/5	
Total station mark	/30	

Learning Points

- A systematic approach to ECG interpretation will help you interpret almost any ECG. Even if there are obvious abnormalities sticking to the system will ensure you don't miss the other more subtle findings.

- ST elevation in 2 or more consecutive ECG leads suggests an acute ST-elevation myocardial infarction. ST elevation must be more than 2 small squares in the chest leads, or more than 1 small square in the limb leads, to be significant.

- Learn your leads;
    Septal leads V1-V2
    Anterior Leads V3-V4
    Lateral Leads V5-V6
    Inferior Leads II, III, aVF

Chest X-Ray

Candidate's Instructions

You are the foundation year doctor in the emergency department. A 42-year old gentleman has been referred to you from his GP with a week's history of cough and worsening shortness of breath.

He has been adequately resuscitated and started on appropriate initial treatment based on clinical findings. You have been asked to chase his chest x-ray and interpret the results.

Interpret the chest x-ray and briefly explain the findings to the patient.

With 2 minutes remaining the examiner will stop you and ask you to summarise your findings and ask you some direct questions.

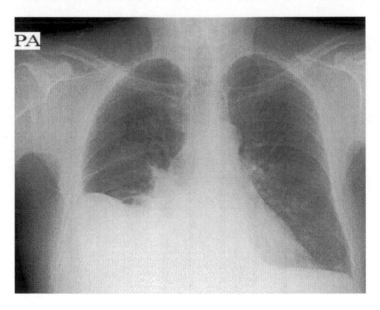

Examiner's Instructions

The candidate is a foundation year doctor in the emergency department seeing a 42-year old gentleman who has presented with a one-week history of productive cough and shortness of breath.

Provide the candidate with a copy of the chest x-ray showing a moderate unilateral pleural effusion. Please ask the candidate to present the chest x-ray to you, and then proceed to explain the findings to the patient.

Please stop the candidate at 6 minutes to discuss further management of pleural effusions.

Actor's Instructions

You are a 42-year-old gentleman. One week ago you developed a cough, and you were bringing up yellow-green sputum. Four days ago, you started feeling short of breath while walking up the stairs and this has been getting worse. You have been feeling hot and sweaty at times.

Your wife was concerned so she took you to the local emergency department, where they have started you on antibiotics and given you a bag of fluids. You still feel uncomfortable breathing, and are waiting for the results of your chest x-ray that was taken an hour ago.

You are otherwise usually well and you don't take any regular medications. You work as a bank manager and smoke 10 cigarettes a day.

You listen carefully to the explanation given by the candidate. You may prompt with questions about the most likely cause and next steps if required. You are happy with the explanation given, and do not have any further questions for the candidate.

Chest X-Ray; pleural effusion

Task:	Achieved	Not Achieved
Interpretation/Presentation of chest x-ray		
Confirms patient details and date		
Comments on the position of the radiograph (AP/PA) film		
Comments on exposure		
Comments on rotation		
Comments on adequacy of field of view		
Comments on inspiratory effort		
Comments on trachea and mediastinum		
Comments on size of heart and cardiac borders		
Comments on costophrenic and cardiophrenic angles		
Comments on lung fields		
Identifies unilateral pleural effusion with meniscus and adjacent opacification.		
Comments on the presence of any extras; oxygen tubing, ECG leads, pacemakers, lines etc.		
Comments on soft tissue and bony abnormalities		
Explanation to patient		
Introduces self and role		
Explains the presence of a pleural effusion		
Briefly explains the likely cause and further management required		
Discussion with examiner		
Identifies parapneumonic effusion as most likely diagnosis		
Able to discuss differential diagnoses		
Identifies need for aspiration		
Adequate discussion on pleural fluid aspirate interpretation		
Examiner's Global Mark	/5	
Actor / Helper's Global Mark	/5	
Total Station Mark	/30	

Learning Points

- When discussing the causes of a pleural effusion, remember to divide causes into transudate and exudate.

- On pleural fluid analysis, if protein < 25g/dl, the effusion is a transudate. If protein > 35g/dl, the effusion is an exudate.

- Light's criteria is applied if the protein content of the pleural fluid is between 25 – 35 g/dl to determine the nature of the fluid.

Abdominal X-ray

Candidate's Instructions

You are the foundation year doctor on call for medicine. You are looking after a 57-year-old man who has been in hospital for the past week being treated for sepsis.

The nurse has asked you to review this patient because he is complaining of abdominal pain and diarrhoea.

You have assessed him and requested an abdominal x-ray. The result is now available. Please interpret the x-ray and discuss your findings with the medical registrar.

With 2 minutes remaining the examiner will stop you and ask you to summarise your findings and ask you some direct questions.

Examiner's Instructions

The candidate has been asked to interpret an abdominal x-ray and discuss it with the medical registrar. The x-ray is of a 57 year old man who has been in hospital for 1 week being treated for sepsis. He is complaining of abdominal pain and has had diarrhoea.

The correct diagnosis is toxic megacolon secondary to clostridium difficile (C.diff).

Please stop the candidate at 6 minutes to discuss further management. Initial investigations may include bloods (inflammatory markers, FBC, UE, LFT, Clotting, lactate), stool cultures and an erect chest x-ray.

Initial management may include ABCDE assessment of the patient, intravenous fluids, electrolyte replacement, bowel rest (NBM), antibiotics (as per microbiology guidelines) and a surgical review.

AXR- toxic megacolon

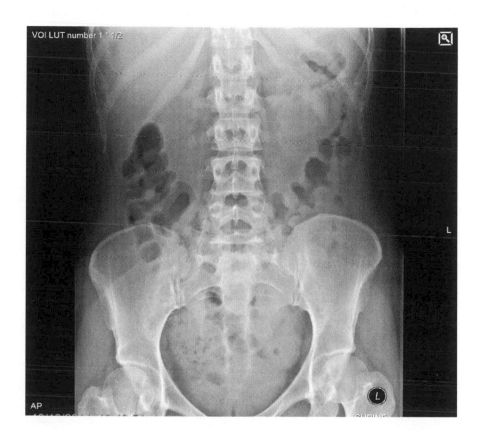

Actor's Instructions

You are the medical registrar on-call. The candidate has requested an abdominal x-ray on a 57-year-old medical patient who is complaining of abdominal pain and diarrhoea. The patient has been in hospital for a week receiving intravenous antibiotics for the treatment of sepsis.

The candidate will present their findings to you.

Abdominal X-ray

Task:	Achieved	Not Achieved
Confirms patient details and date		
Comments on x-ray position (supine, lateral decubitus)		
Comments on x-ray quality		
Comments on exposure		
Comments on rotation		
Identifies small bowel (valvulae conniventes, central position, <3cm)		
Identifies large bowel (haustra, peripheral location)		
Comments on obvious abnormality		
Correctly identifies large bowel is enlarged (>6cm)		
Identifies thumbprinting		
Looks for abnormalities of the soft tissues		
Looks for abnormalities of the solid organs		
Looks for bony abnormalities		
Looks for evidence of bowel perforation		
Looks for evidence of stones or calcific abnormalities		
Presents findings in concise logical manner		
Discussion with examiner		
Gives appropriate differential diagnosis		
Gives correct diagnosis – toxic megacolon		
Gives appropriate list of investigations		
Gives appropriate management plan		
Examiner's Global Mark	/5	
Actor / Helper's Global Mark	/5	
Total Station Mark	/30	

Learning Points

- Toxic megacolon is a life-threatening complication of inflammatory or infectious colitis.

- In this case C.diff infection secondary to antibiotics is the most likely cause. C. difficile infections can be caused by fluoroquinolones, cephalosporins, clindamycin and penicillins and should be considered in any patient who has recently received antibiotics with new onset diarrhoea or abdominal pain.

- If the patient shows signs of worsening toxicity, (progressive dilatation, evidence of perforation or haemorrhage) then surgery should be considered.

Type 2 Respiratory Failure

Candidate's Instructions

You are the foundation year doctor on call for the medical wards. You are bleeped to see Joe a 60-year-old man with COPD who has become increasingly drowsy and breathless.

As part of your initial ABC assessment, you perform an arterial blood gas. Interpret the ABG result given to you and present your findings to the examiner.

Examiner's Instructions

Joe is a 60-year-old man with known COPD has become drowsy on the respiratory ward.

The foundation doctor on call has been bleeped to review the patient. As part of an ABCDE assessment an arterial blood gas has been done. The actor/helper (nurse) has run the gas and presents the printout of results to the candidate. The ABG shows a decompensated chronic type 2 respiratory failure.

Encourage the candidate to take a few minutes to look at the ABG result and interpret it. When the candidate is ready, ask them to present their findings. Prompt the candidate to state if the picture is compensated or decompensated. Ask the candidate to summarise the next steps in the management of this patient. Ask for common causes for type 2 respiratory failure – commonest cause: COPD, others: reduced respiratory effort (e.g. drug effect), chest wall deformity.

If time allows and if candidate is doing well, ask the candidate to explain the difference between type 1 and type 2 respiratory failure.

Actor's Instructions

You are a nurse and have just started on shift. You are looking after Joe a 60-year-old man with COPD who has become increasingly drowsy. You run the ABG for the foundation doctor on call and give him/her the print out. The patient is not on any oxygen. If candidate asks you about the patient's history, say, "I'm not sure, sorry" and do not provide any additional information.

ABG Print out

Patient:	Joe					
FiO$_2$:	21%					
Sample:	Arterial					

Blood Gas Values							
pH	**7.293**		[	7.350	-	7.450	]
pCO$_2$	**9.00**	kPa	[	4.00	-	6.50	]
pO$_2$	**7.2**	kPa	[	12.0	-	15.0	]
Acid Base Status							
HCO$_3^-$	**32**	mmol/L	[	22	-	28	]
BE	**8.9**	mmol/L	[	-3.0	-	3.0	]
Oximetry Values							
Hb	**135**	g/L	[	135	-	175	]
SaO$_2$	**84.0**	%	[	95.0	-	100.0	]
Electrolyte Values							
K$^+$	**4.2**	mmol/L	[	3.5	-	5.0	]
Na$^+$	**137**	mmol/L	[	135	-	145	]
ion Ca^{2+}	**1.15**	mmol/L	[	1.10	-	1.35	]
Cl$^-$	**102**	mmol/L	[	96	-	106	]
Anion Gap	**3.0**	mmol/L	[	8.0	-	16.0	]
Metabolic Values							
Lact	**1.0**	mmol/L	[	0.5	-	2.0	]
Bili	**6**	μmol/L	[		-		]

Type 2 Respiratory Failure

Task:	Achieved	Not Achieved
Confirms patient details on printout are correct – name, date of birth and hospital number		
Confirms whether patient was on oxygen at time ABG taken		
Looks at the pH		
Identifies whether normal/ acidotic/ alkalotic		
Looks at pCO_2		
Identifies whether low/normal/high		
Looks at pO2		
Identifies whether low/normal/ high		
Looks at the bicarbonate		
Identifies whether low/normal/ high		
Looks at the BE		
Identifies whether low/normal/ high		
Looks at the lactate		
Identifies whether low/normal/ high		
Comments on electrolytes		
Comments on haemoglobin		
Presents findings in concise, logical manner		
Discusses management of patient		
Discusses causes of type 2 respiratory failure		
Discusses difference between type 1 and type 2 respiratory failure		
Examiner's Global Mark	/5	
Actor / Helper's Global Mark	/5	
Total Station Mark	/30	

Learning Points

- Always double check patient identifiers first to make sure you are reviewing results of the right patient.

- Check whether the patient was on oxygen or not (and how much) as this may affect your interpretation of the pO_2 and ABG.

- Practice and develop a methodical approach to ABGs so you can recognize patterns quickly and present in a confident manner.

Look first at the **pH**

Then at the **pCO$_2$**

Then at the **pO$_2$**

Then at the **bicarbonate** and **base excess**

Then at the **lactate**

Type 1 Respiratory Failure

Candidate's Instructions

You are the foundation year doctor on call for the medical wards. You are asked to review the progress of a young lady called Sam with an exacerbation of asthma and review a repeat arterial blood gas that the nurse has done for you.

Interpret the ABG result given to you and present your findings to the examiner.

Examiner's Instructions

Sam is a 20-year-old lady with asthma who has been admitted via the emergency department with an acute exacerbation. She was extremely tachypnoeic on admission and required treatment with steroids, back-to-back nebulisers and magnesium sulphate. An initial gas on admission showed a respiratory alkalosis with hypoxia.

The candidate has been asked to review the progress of this young lady and interpret a repeat arterial blood gas that the nurse has performed. The patient initially stabilized with treatment, but over the past hour has deteriorated. She is now tachypnoeic, engaging accessory muscles and looking fatigued.

Encourage the candidate to take a few minutes to review and interpret the result. When the candidate is ready ask them to present their findings. Prompt the candidate to identify the type of respiratory failure if required.

Once the candidate has identified the abnormalities ask the candidate how they would like to manage the patient, the causes of type 1 respiratory failure and the difference between type 1 respiratory failure.

Actor's Instructions

You are the nurse on the medical ward. You are looking after a 20-year-old lady who has been admitted with an exacerbation of asthma. The emergency department handed over that she came in with a severe exacerbation requiring back-to-back nebulisers, steroids and intravenous magnesium sulphate. When you first took over she was settled, but over the past hour she has become increasingly tachypnoeic, is using accessory muscles to breath and is starting to look fatigued.

You are concerned about this patient. You have done an ABG and called the foundation doctor Give him or her the print out.

If they ask, observations are as follows;
RR30, Sats 94%, FiO_2 30%, HR 120, BP 110/70, Temp 36.5

ABG Print out:

Patient:	Sam							
FiO$_2$:	30%							
Sample:	Arterial							
Blood Gas Values								
pH	**7.451**			[	7.350	-	7.450	]
pCO$_2$	**4.50**	kPa		[	4.00	-	6.50	]
pO$_2$	**8.4**	kPa		[	12.0	-	15.0	]
Acid Base Status								
HCO$_3^-$	**23**	mmol/L		[	22	-	28	]
BE	**-2.6**	mmol/L		[	-3.0	-	3.0	]
Oximetry Values								
Hb	**135**	g/L		[	135	-	175	]
SaO$_2$	**94.0**	%		[	95.0	-	100.0	]
Electrolyte Values								
K$^+$	**4.2**	mmol/L		[	3.5	-	5.0	]
Na$^+$	**137**	mmol/L		[	135	-	145	]
ion Ca^{2+}	**1.15**	mmol/L		[	1.10	-	1.35	]
Cl$^-$	**102**	mmol/L		[	96	-	106	]
Anion Gap	**12.0**	mmol/L		[	8.0	-	16.0	]
Metabolic Values								
Lact	**1.0**	mmol/L		[	0.5	-	2.0	]
Bili	**6**	μmol/L		[		-		]

Type 1 Respiratory Failure

Task:	Achieved	Not Achieved
Confirms patient details on printout are correct – name, date of birth and hospital number		
Confirms whether patient was on oxygen at time ABG taken		
Looks at the pH		
Identifies whether normal/ acidotic/ alkalotic		
Looks at pCO_2		
Identifies whether low/normal/high		
Looks at pO2		
Identifies whether low/normal/ high		
Looks at the bicarbonate		
Identifies whether low/normal/ high		
Looks at the BE		
Identifies whether low/normal/ high		
Looks at the lactate		
Identifies whether low/normal/ high		
Comments on electrolytes		
Comments on haemoglobin		
Presents findings in concise, logical manner		
Discusses management of patient		
Discusses causes of type 1 respiratory failure		
Discusses difference between type 1 and type 2 respiratory failure		
Examiner's Global Mark	/5	
Actor / Helper's Global Mark	/5	
Total Station Mark	/30	

Learning Points

- Always interpret an ABG in the context of the patient's clinical condition. In this case a rising CO2 in an asthmatic patient who is tachypnoeic, working hard and tiring is a worrying sign suggesting the patient may need intubation and ventilation.

- As a general rule;

$$FiO2-10=paO_2$$

i.e. the arterial oxygenation concentration should be interpreted in the context of how much oxygen is being given to the patient. If there is a mismatch between the expected and the measured paO2, this suggests the patient is "relatively hypoxaemic" for the amount of oxygen delivered

- Don't forget to look at the lactate, Hb and electrolytes as this may provide you with important clues.

Metabolic Acidosis (DKA)

Candidate's Instructions

You are the foundation year doctor on call for the acute medical admissions unit. You have been asked to assess Lucy a 29-year old lady who has been admitted with abdominal pain and drowsiness.

As part of your initial ABCDE assessment, you perform an arterial blood gas. Please interpret the ABG result provided and present your findings to the examiner.

Examiner's Instructions

Lucy a 29-year-old lady with known type 1 diabetes has been admitted to the ward with abdominal pain and drowsiness. The patient is restless and appears unwell from the end of the bed.

The foundation doctor on call has been bleeped to review the patient. As part of an ABCDE assessment an arterial blood gas has been done. The actor/helper (nurse) has run the gas and presents the printout of results to the candidate.

Encourage the candidate to take a few minutes to look at the ABG result and interpret it. When the candidate is ready, ask them to present their findings. Prompt the candidate to identify the type of acidosis and to give a diagnosis.

If at this point the candidate is struggling, please inform them the gas shows diabetic ketoacidosis. This piece of information is important in order for them to proceed with the station. Ask the candidate the diagnostic criteria for DKA and how they would like to manage this patient.

Actor's instructions

You are the nurse looking after Lucy a 29-year old lady who has become increasingly unwell on the ward. You run the ABG for the FY1 on call and give him/her the print out. The patient had this ABG done on air. You can tell the candidate this if they ask you.

If candidate tries to ask you about the patient's history, say, "I'm not sure, sorry" and do not provide any additional information.

ABG Print out:

Patient:		Lucy					
FiO_2:	21%						
Sample:	Arterial						
Blood Gas Values							
pH	7.290			[	7.350	-	7.450
pCO_2	3.40	kPa		[	4.00	-	6.50
pO_2	11.8	kPa		[	12.0	-	15.0
Acid Base Status							
HCO_3^-	12	mmol/L		[	22	-	28
BE	-11.0	mmol/L		[	-3.0	-	3.0
Oximetry Values							
Hb	135	g/L		[	135	-	175
SaO_2	98.9	%		[	95.0	-	100.0
Electrolyte Values							
K^+	3.0	mmol/L		[	3.5	-	5.0
Na^+	138	mmol/L		[	135	-	145
ion Ca^{2+}	1.15	mmol/L		[	1.10	-	1.35
Cl^-	82	mmol/L		[	96	-	106
Anion Gap	44.0	mmol/L		[	8.0	-	16.0
Metabolic Values							
Lact	1.0	mmol/L		[	0.5	-	2.0
Gluc	20	mmol/L			4	-	6

Metabolic Acidosis (DKA)

Task:	Achieved	Not Achieved
Confirms patient details on printout are correct – name, date of birth and hospital number		
Confirms whether patient was on oxygen at time ABG taken		
Looks at the pH		
Identifies whether normal/ acidotic/ alkalotic		
Looks at pCO_2		
Identifies whether low/normal/high		
Looks at pO2		
Identifies whether low/normal/ high		
Looks at the bicarbonate		
Identifies whether low/normal/ high		
Looks at the BE		
Identifies whether low/normal/ high		
Looks at the lactate		
Identifies whether low/normal/ high		
Comments on electrolytes		
Comments on haemoglobin		
Presents findings in concise, logical manner		
Makes diagnosis of metabolic acidosis with respiratory compensation secondary to DKA		
Discusses management of patient		
Discusses diagnostic criteria of DKA		
Examiner's Global Mark	/5	
Actor / Helper's Global Mark	/5	
Total Station Mark	/30	

Learning Points

- It is essential to know the diagnostic criteria for diabetic ketoacidosis:
    - Blood glucose > 11.0mmol/L or known diabetes mellitus
    - Ketonaemia > 3.0mmol/L or significant ketonuria (more than 2+ on standard urine sticks)
    - Bicarbonate (HCO3-) < 15.0mmol/L and/or venous pH < 7.3

- In the management of DKA you should always take an ABCDE approach. In the first hour of management fluid resuscitation and a fixed rate insulin infusion are the mainstay of management.

- In DKA it is important to remember that initially serum potassium is often normal or high but total body potassium is low and hypokalaemia can be fatal. In view of this close monitoring and potassium replacement are essential.

Alcohol Excess

Candidate's Instructions

You are the medical foundation year doctor on call. You have been asked to see James a 32-year-old gentleman, with generalised abdominal pain and vomiting. On examination, he appears sweaty and has a tremor. James would like to know the results of his blood tests taken earlier today. Please interpret the following results, summarising and discuss your findings with the patient. Discuss the likely causes and suggest further management.

BLOOD RESULTS

Patient Name: James
DOB: 15/05/1984
Hospital No: M1234567

Hb	131
MCV	106
PLT	118
WCC	4.7
Na	132 mmol/l
K	3.2 mmol/l
Urea	2.5 mmol/l
Creatinine	58 µmol/l
Albumin	30 g/l
AST	34 IU/l
ALT	33 IU/l
GGT	139 IU/l
Bilirubin	11 µmol/l
ALP	65U/l

Examiner's Instructions

The candidate is the medical foundation doctor on call. James is a 32-year-old patient, with generalised abdominal pain and vomiting. He has been asking for the results of his blood tests that were taken earlier today. The candidate has been asked to explain the findings of these results to the patient, exploring with him the causes for these abnormalities and deciding on a management plan with the patient.

The candidate must take a brief history, explain that the blood results show changes consistent with excess alcohol intake and formulate a management plan with the patient.

Actor's Instructions

You are a 32-year-old banker working in the city. You have been under a lot of stress working on a busy project over the past 8 months. This has involved several late nights at work to meet your deadlines, usually followed by a few drinks at the local public house. Your current alcohol consumption is in excess, comprising of one or two glasses of wine at lunch or business meetings, and another three pints of beer/cider after every night after work and most weekends, totalling on average 70 units per week (guidelines state weekly intake should not exceed more than 14 units for men and women).

Over the past few weeks you have been getting worsening generalised abdominal pains, dull in nature, but constant at a severity of 6/10 with associated vomiting. You have noticed that you are a bit shaky in the mornings but feel much better after your first drink at lunchtime. You have not had an alcoholic drink for the past two days and have not been eating, as you cannot keep anything down.

You have had your appendix removed but otherwise have no other medical conditions and are not on any regular medications. You have no known drug allergies. You have no family history of alcoholism, but your father had bowel cancer, and is now in remission. You live alone in a flat in the city. You do not take any recreational drugs.

You last had your bloods taken at the age of 14 when your appendix was removed. You smoke 5 cigarettes a day for the past 10 years. You are aware that your alcohol intake is excessive and are willing to cut down. You are concerned that your boss will find out and that you will lose your job.

Alcohol Excess

Task:	Achieved:	Not achieved:
Introduces self		
Checks name and DOB with patient		
Consents patient for discussion		
Checks understanding of why tests have been done		
Elicits any patient concerns		
Ask when bloods were last taken		
Explains that routine blood tests were taken to help determine the cause for his symptoms.		
Explains some of these results are abnormal, therefore you would like to ask a few further questions		
Checks for symptoms of alcohol excess/withdrawal		
Asks about past medical history, medications and allergies, family history and social history		
Explores cause: asks about alcohol intake and quantifies units		
CAGE questionnaire		
Explains that the blood tests show changes in particular affecting the markers for liver function		
Explains that these changes are likely due to excessive alcohol consumption and that bowel cancer is an unlikely cause		
Explains that the patient is experiencing withdrawal symptoms		
Explains that the patient will need to cut down on alcohol intake. Asks whether willing to do so and whether would require any help		
Explains that we will give medication to help with withdrawal symptoms and to replenish losses in any vitamins/minerals/fluids which commonly occurs with excess alcohol consumption		
Close		
Summarises discussion		
Checks understanding and answers any questions		
Thanks patient		

Examiner's Global Mark	/5	
Actor / Helper's Global Mark	/5	
Total Station Mark	/30	

Learning points

- Use a structured approach when faced with data interpretation stations (e.g. Introduction, History, Explanation of Data, Management Plan)

- A brief history from the patient in these stations as may give you clues about the cause if you are unclear from the results alone

- Remember to explore the patient's concerns and reassure them where necessary

Pseudogout

Candidate's Instructions

You are a foundation year doctor in the emergency department. You have been asked to see Ethel an 82-year-old female with an acutely swollen left knee. Joint aspiration was performed showing a raised white cell count, predominantly neutrophils, and intra- and extracellular weakly positive birefringent crystals.

Please take a brief history from this patient, review the results of her joint aspiration, explain the likely diagnosis and formulate a management plan.

Examiner's Instructions

The candidate is a foundation doctor in the emergency department. Ethel Jones is an 82-year-old female who has presented with a fever and an acutely swollen left knee. Joint aspiration of small effusion surrounding the knee was performed to rule out a septic arthritis, revealing weakly positive birefringent crystals. The candidate must take a brief history from the patient, interpret and explain the results to the patient and formulate a management plan for pseudogout.

Actor's Instructions

You are Ethel, an 82-year-old female, presenting to the emergency department today with an acutely swollen left knee. You developed pain in the left knee yesterday evening but put this down to old age. This morning when you woke up, you were unable to bear weight on your left leg due to pain in the left knee and almost fell over. You noticed that the knee was red, warm to touch and swollen. You have been feeling hot and cold for the last two days, waking up in the night and finding your pillow drenched with sweat. You have also had slight loss of appetite and have not been eating or drinking as much as you normally do. You are afraid to stand as you do not want to fall. You are concerned that you not be able to walk again and look after your husband who has Alzheimer's. You insist that you are told the results before a history is taken but back down once reassured by the doctor that taking a history first will help to put these results into context.

Your past medical history includes hypertension, Type 2 Diabetes mellitus and hypothyroidism. You take Amlodipine, Metformin, Simvastatin and Levothyroxine. You are allergic to penicillin, which gave you a widespread rash as a child. You have no significant family history.

You live with your husband in a bungalow. You do not have any carers. You have a daughter who lives nearby and helps with the shopping, cleaning and meals. You mobilise with a stick. You have never smoked and drink a glass of bubbly on special occasions only.

Pseudogout

Task:	Achieved:	Not achieved:
Introduces self		
Checks name and DOB with patient		
Consents patient for discussion		
Checks understanding of why tests have been done and cause for symptoms		
Elicits any concerns		
Explains that fluid was taken from the joint to rule out an infection and find the cause for her symptoms		
Explains that before discussing the results that you'd like to ask a few questions		
Explains that you understand that patient would like to know the results beforehand but by taking a history first, this will help to put their results into context		
Elicits symptoms: red, warm to touch, painful, unable to weightbear, fever		
Explores past medical history		
Asks for list of regular medications and drug allergies		
Asks about family history and social history, including briefly assessing functional status (mobility etc.)		
Explains that fluid result shows crystals		
Explains that diagnosis is pseudogout		
Explains that mainstay of treatment is ice packs, rest, anti-inflammatory medication and in some cases steroid injections		
Assesses for contraindications to NSAIDs or steroids		
Explains that likely to resolve within 10 days but may cause long term functional limitation		
Summarises discussion		
Checks understanding and answers any questions		
Thanks patient		
Examiner's Global Mark	/5	
Actor / Helper's Global Mark	/5	
Total Station Mark	/30	

Learning points

- Use a structured approach when faced with data interpretation stations (e.g. Introduction, History, Explanation of Data, Management Plan)

- Remember to consider and rule in/out the most important diagnosis – septic arthritis – in an acutely, red, hot, swollen joint

- Don't forget to consider treatment alternatives if the patient has any contraindications (e.g. Colchicine if cannot take steroids or NSAIDs in this case)

Pleural Fluid

Candidate's Instructions

While working on a respiratory ward, the consultant asks you to look at the results of a pleural fluid sample. It was recently taken from Herbert a patient who was diagnosed with a pleural effusion. Please look at the pleural fluid results below and interpret accordingly:

Pleural Fluid Pathology Report

Patient name: Herbert

Sample taken 05/09/16 at 14:30

Appearance: cloudy, straw coloured fluid

Biochemistry
Total protein: 32 g/L
Glucose: 3.3 mmol/L (LOW)
pH: 7.35
Amylase: not raised

Pleural fluid protein/serum protein: 0.8
Pleural fluid LDH/serum: LDH 0.7
Pleural fluid LDH: normal

Microbiology
Gram stain: no organisms seen

Cytology
No malignant cells seen

Please explain the results and further management to Herbert.

Examiner's Instructions

You are the consultant on the respiratory ward and you have asked the junior doctor to look at the results from a pleural fluid sample from Herbert a patient diagnosed with a pleural effusion. They have been asked to interpret the results and explain the results to the patient

Due to the borderline level of protein in the sample (32g/L) the candidate should use Light's criteria using the values listed to confirm the sample is an **exudate.** If the candidate fails to identify the sample is an exudate, please tell them this as it is essential for them to be able to complete the rest of the station.

There are no other diagnostic features from this sample to help narrow the differential diagnosis. They should explain to the patient that further investigations to establish a cause for the pleural effusion may be required. These may include a CT scan of the thorax and abdomen, or a VATS (video assisted thorascopic surgery) and biopsy procedure.

At 6 minutes stop the candidate and ask them to list 3 causes of a transudate and 3 causes of an exudate. Ask them to describe Light's criteria and when it is used.

Transudate	Exudate
Heart failure	Infection
Hypoalbuminaemia (liver cirrhosis, nephrotic syndrome)	Inflammation
Hypothyroidism	Infarction (PE)
Peritoneal dialysis	Malignancy
	Tuberculosis
	Connective tissues disorders

Light's Criteria
Fluid is an exudate if one of the following criteria are met;
- Efusion protein:serum ratio >0.5
- Efusion lactate:serum lactate ratio >0.6
- Pleural fluid lactate >2/3 times the upper limit of normal serum LDH

Pleural Fluid

Task:	Achieved:	Not achieved:
Confirms patient age and DOB on sample report		
Confirms time and date on sample report		
Comments on the appearance of the sample		
Comments on the protein level of the sample		
Recognises the need to use Light's criteria due to the borderline protein level		
Uses Light's criteria to determine the sample is an exudate		
Comments on the fluid pH (within normal range)		
Comments on the fluid glucose (low)		
Comments on the gram stain		
Comments on the fluid white cell count		
Comments on the fluid cytology report		
Establishes patient's understanding of condition and tests undertaken		
Elicits any patient concerns		
Explains to patient that the result has shown the that the pleural fluid is protein rich		
Explains to the patient that currently the cause for the pleural effusion is unclear and that there are several differentials		
Explains to the patient that further investigations to establish the cause of the effusion may be required		
Answers the patient's questions		
Able to list 3 causes of a transudate		
Able to list 3 causes of an exudate		
Able to describe Light's criteria and it's use		
Examiner's Global Mark	/5	
Actor / Helper's Global Mark	/5	
Total Station Mark	/30	

Learning Points

- Serous pleural fluid can be classed as either transudate or exudate by looking at protein value.

- Light's criteria should be used when protein value is borderline (25-35g/L). One or more of the three criteria must be positive to confirm sample is an exudate.

- Common causes for exudate pleural fluids include infection, malignancy, inflammation, and infarction.

Clinical Skills

Manual BP Measurement

Candidate's instructions

A 65-year-old man was seen in clinic for hypertension and started on some new medication to lower his blood pressure. He has returned to the GP practice today to get it rechecked.

The GP has asked you to check his blood pressure using a manual machine. Please explain your findings to the patient.

Examiner's Instructions

A 65-year-old man was seen in clinic for hypertension and started on some new medications. He has returned to the GP practice today to get is rechecked.

The candidate is a foundation doctor. They have been asked by the GP to check this gentleman's blood pressure using a manual machine. The candidate should check the blood pressure first by feeling the pulse as an estimate, then by auscultating the artery. They should then explain their findings to the patient.

At 6 minutes stop the candidate and ask them to present their findings and explain the clinical significance.

Actor's Instructions

You have recently been diagnosed with high blood pressure and started on some medication. You have been taking your medications every day. You have returned to the GP practice today to get your blood pressure rechecked.

You have been quite worried about the diagnosis of high blood pressure. Your father had high blood pressure and eventually suffered stroke. You were told the high blood pressure may have been a contributing factor.

You are anxious to know the result of the repeat blood pressure measurement.

Manual Blood Pressure Measurement

Task:	Achieved	Not Achieved
Wash hands		
Introduces self and clarifies patients' details		
Explains procedure and gains informed consent		
Asks the patient if they have any pain		
Ensure patient positioned comfortably		
Assembles equipment		
Select the correct size cuff		
Wrap cuff around arm with arrow aligned with brachial artery		
Palpates brachial artery		
Inflate cuff and estimates systolic blood pressure		
Fully deflates cuff		
Inflates cuff to above estimated figure whilst auscultating the artery		
Deflates cuff slowly		
Notes reading at which first Korotkoff sound heard		
Notes the value when Korotkoff sound disappears		
Fully deflates cuff		
Thanks patient and informs of reading		
Informs patient of management required (i.e. continue current medications, up-titrate dose)		
Advise of follow up		
Presents findings and clinical significance in a clear, concise, logical manner		
Examiner's Global Mark	/5	
Actor / Helper's Global Mark	/5	
Total Station Mark	/27	

Learning Points

- Blood pressure measurements with an automated device in patients with an irregular pulse may be inaccurate. In these circumstances a manual blood pressure is required.

- Cuff size is very important. If it is too small the blood pressure reading will be falsely elevated. If the cuff is too large the blood pressure reading will be artificially low. The blood pressure cuffs have sizing guides on them to help guide your choice.

- In patients <80 years the target blood pressure is <140/90mmHg, and for patients >80 years the target blood pressure is <150/90mmHg. Blood pressure targets for those with CKD and Diabetes will be different.

NG Tube Insertion

Candidate's Instructions

You are the foundation doctor on the acute stroke ward. Rita is an 85 year old lady who has had difficulty swallowing after a right hemispheric ischaemic stroke. The Speech and Language Team have recommended an NG tube for feeding.

You have been asked by the nursing team to insert the nasogastric tube. Please demonstrate on the model provided.

Examiner's Instructions

The foundation doctor on the acute stroke ward has been asked to insert a nasogastric tube. Rita is an 85 year old lady who presented with a right hemispheric ischaemic stroke and has swallowing difficulties. She has been assessed by the speech and language team and has an unsafe swallow. They have recommended an NG tube for feeding.

Please assess their technique. A model will be provided.

Actor's Instructions

You are Rita. An 85-year-old lady who has had an ischaemic stroke affecting the left hand side of your body. It has not affected your speech, but you are having difficulties swallowing. The Speech and Language therapist thinks your swallow is unsafe and has recommended and NG tube for feeding.

You have not had an NG tube before and are apprehensive about the procedure and whether it will cause any pain.

The candidate will demonstrate the correct procedure on the manikin provided.

NG Tube Insertion

Task:	Achieved:	Not achieved:
Washes hands		
Introduces Self and clarifies patients' details		
Explains procedure and gains informed consent		
Establishes any contraindications to the procedure		
Asks the patient if they have any pain		
Positions patient in the upright position		
Assembles equipment (Trolley, Apron, Non-sterile gloves, Ryles Tube, KY jelly, dressing, adhesive tape, bladder syringe, receptacle, pH paper)		
Puts on apron and non-sterile gloves		
Correctly measures length of NG tube (ear-lobe to tip of nose to xiphisternum)		
Lubricates tip of NG tube		
Inserts NG tube into nostril		
Gently advances tube through nasopharynx		
Asks patient to mimic swallow to ease passage of NG tube		
Advances NG tube to estimated length.		
Fixes tube with adhesive tape and dressing		
Removes guidewire and disposes in sharps pin		
Aspirates gastric contents with bladder syringe		
Tests pH of aspirated contents and comments on whether the tube is safe to use		
Thanks patient		
Documents procedure clearly		
Examiner's Global Mark	/5	
Actor / Helper's Global Mark	/5	
Total Station Mark	/30	

Learning Points

- An aspirate with a pH <5.5 means that the tube is in the stomach, and it is safe to use. If the aspirate is > pH 6 the tube should not be used. The aspirate should be repeated in an hour, and if there remains any doubt about the tube position a CXR should be obtained to confirm position.

- If you are unable to obtain an aspirate various manoeuvres may help such as providing mouth care, advancing the tube by 1-2cm or lying the patient in the left lateral position Asking the patient to mimic a swallow, tilt their chin down or taking a sip of water (if safe to do so) may help pass the NG tube into the oesophagus.

- Misplaced NG tubes have been deemed a 'never event' in the NHS'. Never Events are serious incidents that are wholly preventable as guidance or safety recommendations that provide strong systemic protective barriers are available at a national level and should have been implemented by all healthcare providers. Other examples of never events include: wrong site surgery and retained instruments post operation.

Ankle Brachial Pulse Index

Candidate Instructions

You are the foundation year doctor working in geriatrics outpatients. Winston, an 85 year old gentleman, has been experiencing calf pain on the left side whilst mobilising.

Please measure an ABPI, on the left hand side only, and document this procedure on the paper provided.

With 2 minutes remaining the examiner will stop you and ask you to summarise your findings and ask you some direct questions.

Examiner's Instructions

The candidate is a foundation year doctor working in geriatrics outpatients. Winston is an 85 year old gentleman who is complaining of progressively worsening calf pain on the left hand side, which is now starting to affect his mobility.

The candidate has been asked to perform an ABPI on the left hand side and document their findings on the paper provided. If the candidate tries to take bilateral measurements please move them on.

At 6 minutes please ask the candidate about their findings and their interpretation of these findings.

Actor's Instructions

You are an 85 year old retired painter who has been experiencing left sided calf pain which has been getting progressively worse over the last six months. Over the last month the pain is present at rest. It is now starting to affect your mobility. You are an ex-smoker with a 40 year pack history. You have T2DM, hypertension and previously had a CABG at aged 65 due to triple vessel disease. You are anxious that you will be told you need an operation.

ABPI

Task:	Achieved:	Not achieved:
Washes hands		
Introduces Self and clarifies patients' details		
Explains procedure and gains informed consent		
Establishes any contraindications to the procedure		
Asks the patient if they have any pain		
Positions patient lying down		
Assembles equipment (Continuous wave doppler unit, ultrasound gel, sphygmomanometer, calculator, non-sterile gloves)		
Places an appropriately sized cuff around the arm		
Locates the brachial pulse and applies ultrasound gel over the skin.		
Correctly holds the probe at a 45 degree angle in the direction of the blood flow in the artery and ensures a good signal		
Inflates the sphygmomanometer cuff until the signal disappears then slowly releases the pressure (22mmHg/second) until the signal returns. Records this value as the brachial systolic pressure.		
States would repeat the above on the other arm.		
Places the same sized cuff around the ankle above the malleoli		
Locates the dorsalis pedis pulse and applies ultrasound gel over the skin. Takes the ankle systolic pressure as described for the brachial and documents the result		
States they would repeat the above for the other ankle.		
Wipes the ultrasound gel from the skin and from the Doppler probe.		
Calculates the ABPI via the following equation: *ABPI= Highest Ankle Doppler pressure (for each leg)/Highest brachial Doppler pressure*		
Interprets the ABPI (>1.0-Normal, 0.4-0.8 Claudication, 0.1-0.4 Critical Ischaemia).		
Thanks patient		
Documents procedure clearly		

Examiner's Global Mark	/5	
Actor / Helper's Global Mark	/5	
Total Station Mark	/30	

Learning Points

- The ratio of arm and ankle systolic pressure (the ABPI), which eliminates systolic pressure variation, is used to assess and monitor peripheral arterial disease. Remember that in patients with diabetes the ABPI can be falsely elevated, and therefore results in these patients should be interpreted with caution.

- Practice co-ordinating inflating the cuff and keeping the Doppler probe in place, this can be tricky.

- Learn the equation for calculating the ABPI and how to interpret the result obtained:

In a normal individual, the ABPI is between 0.92 and 1.3 with the majority of people having a ratio between 1 and 1.2.

An ABPI above 1.3 is usually indicative of non-compressible blood vessels.

An ABPI <0.9 indicates some arterial disease.

An ABPI >0.5 and <0.9 may be associated with intermittent claudication. Refer to a vascular surgeon if symptoms indicate.

An ABPI <0.5 indicates severe arterial disease and may be associated with rest pain, ischaemic ulceration or gangrene and may warrant urgent referral to a vascular surgeon.

Male catheterisation

Candidate's instructions

You are the foundation year doctor on-call for medicine. A 55 year old gentleman has been admitted with severe sepsis and you have been asked to insert a catheter as part of the "Sepsis 6" care bundle to monitor his urine output.

With 2 minutes remaining the examiner will stop you and ask you to summarise your findings and ask you some direct questions.

Examiner's instructions

A 55 year old man has been admitted with severe sepsis and requires catheterisation as part of the "Sepsis 6" care bundle. The on-call medical foundation doctor has been asked to insert a catheter for fluid balance monitoring purposes.

If the candidate requests a chaperone please say that you will chaperone them.

If the candidate pauses to allow time for the anaesthetic lubricant to work please tell them that 5 minutes has elapsed and asked them to proceed.

At 6 minutes please ask the candidate to stop and summarise the main points they would summarise in the patient's notes.

Actor's instructions

You are a 55 year old man who came into hospital very unwell with an infection. You understand that you are very unwell. The nurse has informed you that you require a catheter so that you can be monitored more closely. However, you are anxious as you have not had this procedure before and are worried that it may be painful. You are reassured if the doctor explains the procedure to you and allays your concerns.

If the candidate asks if you would like a chaperone please say yes.

If the candidate asks you whether your penis feels numb after the administration of anaesthetic lubricant and they have allowed a period of time to elapse then tell them it is fine to proceed.

Male Catheterisation

Task	Achieved	Not Achieved
Introduces self to patient		
Explains reason for procedure		
Gains verbal consent		
Reassures patient and answers any questions		
Requests chaperone		
Ensures they have the correct equipment; catheter (14-16Fr), catheter pack, catheter bag, anaesthetic lubricant, saline, gauze, sterile gloves)		
Opens catheter pack and places equipment in the sterile field using an aseptic non-touch technique		
Washes hands and puts on sterile gloves		
Asks patient to expose groin and positions sterile drape		
Retracts foreskin and cleans penis		
Discards gloves, washes hands and puts on a new pair of sterile gloves		
Holds penis using gauze sling and administers anaesthetic lubricant		
Allows at least 5 minutes for anaesthetic lubricant to work		
Holds catheter in the plastic sleeve and inserts catheter into the urethral meatus, advancing it to the hilt.		
Ensure urine is draining before using 10mls of water to inflate the balloon.		
Slowly withdraw catheter until resistance is felt		
Attach the catheter bag		
Retract the patient's foreskin		
Covers the patient and maintains dignity		
States they would document the size of catheter, insertion details, complications, residual volume and colour of urine drained.		
Examiner's Global mark	/5	
Actor's Global mark	/5	
Total station mark	/30	

Learning points

- Ensure that you use aseptic non-touch technique (ANTT) and maintain your sterile field throughout this procedure.

- Ensure that you retract the foreskin post procedure to prevent the development of paraphimosis; this is a urological emergency of allowed to evolve and thus it is good practice to document that you have done this.

- If it is difficult to pass the catheter past the prostate asking the patient to cough, or using a bigger (not smaller) catheter may help.

Setting up a Syringe Driver

Candidate's Instructions

You have been asked to set up a syringe driver for a palliative patient on your ward who is struggling with pain and can no longer to take medications by mouth. The patient already has a subcutaneous butterfly needle in situ.

On the advice of the palliative care team your colleague has prescribed;

5mg diamorphine over 24 hours
10mls water for injection

Please set up and start the syringe driver. Paper and a calculator are provided for you if needed for workings out. There is a nurse available to help you.

Examiner's Instructions

The candidate has been asked to set up a syringe driver for a palliative care patient on the ward who is no longer able to take medications by mouth. The main symptom control issue for this patient is pain. The patient already has a subcutaneous butterfly needle in situ.

A colleague has prescribed the following, on the advice of the palliative care team;

5mg diamorphine over 24 hours
10mls water for injection

Note: 5mg of diamorphine is 1 ampule

There will be approximately 21mls in the syringe to be given over 24 hours, therefore the correct rate is 0.88 mls an hour

Paper and a calculator are provided for the candidate if needed for workings out. A nurse is available to double check drugs, fluids and calculations.

Actor's Instructions

You are a nurse working on the ward. The candidate has been asked to set up a syringe driver with the following prescription;

5mg diamorphine over 24 hours
10mls water for injection

The patient is no longer able to take oral medications, and has pain control issues. The patient already has a subcutaneous needle in-situ that is clean and within date and safe to use. Please assist the candidate by double checking drugs, fluids and calculations with them.

Setting up a Syringe Driver

Task	Achieved	Not Achieved
Washes Hands		
Introduces self		
Confirms patient name, DOB and hospital number		
Explains procedure and gains consent		
Checks prescription on the drug chart		
Checks for drug allergies		
Checks water for injection with helper		
Draw up 20mls water for injection using a syringe and needle (non-touch technique)		
Takes vial of medication prescribed and checks drug, expiry date and concentration with helper (completing controlled drug book)		
Draws up diamorphine into syringe containing water for injection (non-touch technique)		
Places label on syringe (drug name, diluent, patient name, date and time infusion set up, signature)		
Attach the giving set to the syringe and prime the line		
Notes the amount of fluid in the syringe (ml or mm)		
Calculates rate of infusion over 24 hours		
Sets rate on pump		
Places syringe in pump		
Checks the butterfly needle is safe to use (surrounding area, date)		
Attaches syringe to butterfly needle		
Starts infusion		
Disposes of waste safely		
Examiner's global mark	/5	
Actor's global mark	/5	
Total station mark	/30	

Learning Points

- When making drug calculations and using controlled drugs always make sure that you check your work with a second competent colleague.

- There are many different brands of syringe driver and they all use different syringes. Familiarise yourself with the machines used in your trust, that are likely to be used in your exams, and ask the nursing staff to show you how they work.

- A subcutaneous infusion can take 3-4 hours to establish a steady state drug level, therefore a stat dose of medication can be given prior to setting up the driver if the patient is symptomatic.

Setting up a nebuliser

Candidate's Instructions

You are the foundation year doctor in the emergency department. A 24 year-old lady has been admitted with an acute asthma exacerbation.

Please set up a nebulizer and administer salbutamol 5mg to the patient. The salbutamol has been prescribed for you by the consultant in triage. They have specified that the nebuliser should be run on oxygen, and have also prescribed this.

Examiner's Instructions

The candidate is a foundation year doctor in the emergency department. A 24 year-old lady has been admitted with an acute severe asthma exacerbation.

The candidate has been asked to set up a nebulizer and administer 5mg of salbutamol and 500 micrograms of ipratropium that has been prescribed by the consultant in triage. The nebuliser should be run on oxygen, and this has also been prescribed.

Actor's Instructions

You are a 24-year-old lady with asthma. You have been admitted to hospital with worsening of your asthma over the last 24 hours. You became quite short of breath and wheezy last night, and you were unable to control your symptoms with your usual inhalers at home (a brown and blue pump). You have had two previous admissions, neither of which required ITU support. You do not have a cough or fever.

Apart from asthma, you have no other medical conditions or allergies.

You have been told that you will be given some nebulized medication.

Setting up a nebulizer

Task:	Achieved	Not Achieved
Washes hands		
Introduces self		
Confirms patient name, DOB and hospital number		
Explains procedure and gains consent		
Checks prescription on the drug chart		
Checks for drug allergies		
Gathers equipment: facemask, chamber, nebule, tubing, nebulizer		
Checks drug in salbutamol nebule against prescription		
Check expiry date on salbutamol nebule		
Checks drug in ipratropium nebule against prescription		
Checks expiry date on ipratropium nebule		
Assembles nebulizer and tubing, and attaches mouthpiece		
Pours nebules into drug chamber appropriately and closes chamber		
Ensures patient is sitting up		
Ensures facemask fits well around face		
Connects tubing to oxygen point on the wall		
Asks the patient to breathe in and out normally		
Explains nebuliser will last approximately 10-15 minutes		
Advises patient how they will know the nebuliser is finished		
Closes encounter appropriately		
Examiner's Global Mark	/5	
Actor / Helper's Global Mark	/5	
Total Station Mark	/30	

Learning Points

- Ensure you are familiar with all the parts of a nebulizer and are confident assembling them. A separate nebuliser mask with chamber attachment is required.

- Be aware of the indications for nebulized medication and some of the common medications that are given in this form.

- Nebulisers can be given through air or through oxygen, but make sure to clarify which before setting up the nebuliser. The oxygen must be prescribed and this will help set the target saturations and thus may help guide this decision.

Drawing up antibiotics

Candidate's Instructions

A patient with suspected chest sepsis has just been admitted to the Acute Medical Unit.

You are the foundation year doctor on the medical team and have been asked to administer antibiotics as part of the Sepsis 6 bundle.

Draw up antibiotics to give to the patient. Your senior colleague has already prescribed the antibiotic on the patient's drug chart. There is a nurse available to help you.

Examiner's Instructions

A patient with suspected chest sepsis has been admitted to the acute medical unit. They require intravenous antibiotics as part of the "Sepsis 6" care bundle.

The candidate is a foundation year doctor on the medical team. They have been asked to draw up and administer intravenous antibiotics that have been appropriately prescribed by a senior colleague.

Assess the candidate's ability to correctly draw up the antibiotics using aseptic non-touch technique.

Actor's Instructions

You are the nurse looking after a septic patient. The candidate is a foundation year doctor and has been asked to draw up antibiotics to administer to the patient. One of the other doctors on the medical team has already prescribed the antibiotics.

When asked by the candidate, crosscheck the antibiotic/diluents dose and expiry date before it is drawn up and counter-sign it on the drug chart. Do not assist the candidate in finding the relevant equipment or tidying up.

Drawing up antibiotics

Task:	Achieved	Not Achieved
Washes Hands		
Checks prescription on drug chart		
Checks for drug allergies		
Gathers equipment needed (tray, giving set, syringes, needles, labels)		
Checks antibiotic name, dose and expiry date		
Asks nurse to cross check details		
Checks diluent including expiry date		
Asks nurse to cross check details		
Cleans rubber bung with alcohol wipe and allows to dry		
Draws up diluent using syringe and needle		
Injects diluent into antibiotic vial		
Mixes until all powder dissolved		
Draws up dissolved antibiotic and adds to bag of diluent		
Disposes of sharps in a safe manner		
Inserts giving set to bag of diluent and antibiotic and primes line		
Labels bag with patient's details, added drug with dose		
Signs and asks nurse to counter-sign		
Correctly disposes of sharps		
Checks patient allergies and hangs antibiotics		
Maintains aseptic non-touch technique throughout		
Examiner's Global Mark	/5	
Actor / Helper's Global Mark	/5	
Total Station Mark	/30	

Learning Points

- Checking the drug and expiry date before drawing up any medication is an important habit to get into; all medications (including fluids) should be crosschecked before administering.

- Intravenous medications should be drawn up and administered using an aseptic non-touch technique.

- It is important to get into the habit of checking the allergy status to prevent drug errors. The drug chart should be checked, and this information should be confirmed with the patient.

Setting Up IV Fluids

Candidate's Instructions

Whilst working in a busy Medical Admissions Unit, a patient becomes unwell with a severely low blood pressure. A senior colleague has prescribed a stat fluid challenge. The nurses are busy so you have decided to set up the infusion yourself. The patient has a working cannula. The examiner is available to help you if required.

Examiner's Instructions

The candidate is a foundation year doctor on the acute medical unit. A stat fluid challenged has been prescribed, by a senior colleague, for a patient with a low blood pressure. The nurses are busy and unable to put up the fluids. The candidate has been asked to hang them themselves.

If the candidate asks you to crosscheck the prescription, dose and fluid please do this, but please do not provide any further assistance.

Actor's Instructions

You are a patient on the Medical Admissions Unit and are attached to a monitor. The team looking after you have noticed that your blood pressure is low and prescribed a fluid challenge. You are feeling unwell, light headed and cold. You do not have any drug allergies. You have a working cannula that is in-date and shows no sign of infection.

Drawing up IV fluids

Task:	Achieved	Not Achieved
Washes Hands		
Introduces self		
Confirms patient name, DOB and hospital number		
Explains procedure and gains consent		
Checks prescription on the drug chart		
Checks drug allergies		
Gathers equipment; tray, fluid, giving set, alcohol wipes, flushes		
Checks fluid type and additives		
Checks fluid expiry date		
Checks appearance of fluid		
Checks integrity of packaging		
Cross checks with examiner		
Opens fluid and giving set onto tray		
Inserts giving set		
Primes line ensuring there are no air bubbles		
Confirms patient identity with patient and wrist band, and cross checks with prescription		
Checks cannula site (phlebitis, suitability)		
Administers flush of normal saline (5-10mls)		
Attaches giving set connecter to cannula		
Signs drug chart to show fluid has been administered		
Examiner's Global Mark	/5	
Actor's Global Mark	/5	
Total Station Mark	/30	

Learning Points

- Always remember to check the type of fluid, additives, appearance of the fluid, expiration date and integrity of the packaging.

- Always remember to confirm the patient identity and check allergy status even when giving intravenous fluids.

- An IV fluid challenge can be used to try and increase a patient's blood pressure. 500mls is often used. In elderly patients or those with heart failure it is safer to use 250mls and titrate to response with these smaller aliquots.

Putting up Blood

Candidate's Instructions

You are the foundation year doctor on the gastroenterology ward. One of your patients has just returned from endoscopy, where they found a bleeding duodenal ulcer, which was clipped and injected. The patient is no longer bleeding, is haemodynamically stable and has a haemoglobin level of 69g/L. 2 units of packed red cells have been prescribed by your senior colleague.

Please check and administer the first unit. A nurse is available to help you. The cannula has a working cannula.

Examiner's Instructions

The candidate is a foundation year doctor on the gastroenterology ward. They have been asked to check and administer a blood transfusion to a patient who has just come back to the ward from endoscopy.

The candidate must safely check and prepare the unit of blood for administration, assisted by the ward nurse.

Towards the end of the station the candidate may require direct questioning regarding frequency of observations during transfusion and time limits for product administration after removal from temperature controlled storage.

Actor's Instructions

You are an experienced gastroenterology nurse who is competent in checking and administering blood products. Following the candidates lead you should check the patient's identity, prescription, and the blood unit label with them.

You have just performed observations on the patient. The patient's pulse rate is 90 beats per minute, blood pressure 110/81 mmHg, respiratory rate 19, and temperature 36.3 degrees centigrade. The patient's cannula is patent and working well.

The porters brought the blood unit to the ward (out of the blood bank fridge) 20 minutes ago. You would like to know what to do if the transfusion takes longer than the prescribed three hours as you are aware of guidance to complete transfusion within four hours of the blood product leaving controlled temperature storage.

Putting up Blood

Task:	Achieved	Not Achieved
Introduces self		
Clarifies Identity of patient: Name		
Clarifies Identity of patient: Date of Birth		
Clarifies Identity of patient: Patient Number		
Cross-checks 3-point identity with prescription chart		
Cross-checks identity with blood product label		
Checks group of blood unit		
Checks expiry date of blood unit		
Performs two-person checks		
Reviews appropriate duration of administration		
Ensures suitable cannula in situ and functioning		
Ensures appropriate blood giving set available (filter giving set)		
Enquires about consent for receiving blood transfusion		
Checks for any allergies		
Visually inspects unit for damage/precipitants		
Requests / asks to review pre-transfusion observations (pulse rate, blood pressure, respiratory rate, temperature)		
Advises set of observations 15 minutes after start of transfusion		
Advises set of observations 60 minutes post-transfusion		
Aware of maximum time for blood to be out of fridge before return to blood bank when asked		
Maintains professional approach with patient and nursing staff		
Examiner's Global Mark	/5	
Actor / Helper's Global Mark	/5	
Total Station Mark	/30	

Learning Points

- Patient identification is a crucial step in safe blood administration. Positive patient identification requires a minimum of 3 patient identifiers including full name, date of birth and unique identifier number (hospital unit number or NHS number).

- The patient requires regular close observation during transfusion to monitor for the development of any transfusion-related complications. Guidance on the frequency of observations and the observation chart can usually be found on the blood prescription chart.

- Packed red cells must be transfused within 4 hours of leaving the blood bank fridge to avoid waste. They can only be returned to the fridge if they have been out for less than 30 minutes.

Venepuncture

Candidate's Instructions

You are the foundation year doctor on a medical ward. The phlebotomist has not been able to bleed one of your patients as they were busy this morning having a wash.

Please take the samples instead. The patient requires an FBC, U&E, Coagulation Screen and G&S.

Demonstrate how you would do so using the equipment provided.

Examiner's Instructions

The candidate is a foundation year doctor on a medical ward. The phlebotomist has not bled one of their patients. They are required to take the samples instead. The patient requires an FBC, U&E, Coagulation Screen and G&S.

The candidate will perform this skill on the dummy arm using the equipment provided. The actor will provide the voice of the patient.

Actor's Instructions

The candidate has been asked to take blood samples from you. The phlebotomist this morning was unable to take the samples as you were busy having a wash.

You have had bloods taken before, and are happy to have these samples taken. You do not have any concerns about the procedure.

Venepuncture

Task:	Achieved:	Not achieved:
Washes hands		
Introduces self		
Confirms patient name, DOB and hospital number		
Gains consent to take bloods		
Positions patient with forearm resting on cushion		
Selects the correct blood bottles and equipment, including sharps bin		
Applies tourniquet		
Selects appropriate vein		
Puts on gloves		
Cleans the area with an alcohol wipe		
Attaches needle to Vacutainer® correctly		
Warns patient to expect 'sharp scratch' or similar		
Retracts skin distally to stabilise vein and inserts needle correctly		
Attaches blood bottles in the correct order and withdraws blood under vacuum		
Releases tourniquet		
Removes needle and immediately disposes of it in the sharps bin		
Applies pressure to venepuncture site and thanks patient		
Mixes samples gently		
Labels containers correctly by hand (or explains how to do so)		
Fills in appropriate blood form (or explains how to do so)		
Examiner's Global Mark	/5	
Actor / Helper's Global Mark	/5	
Total Station Mark	/30	

Learning points

- It is important to know the correct order of draw; blue (coagulation screen), yellow (U&E), purple (FBC) and then pink (G&S) bottles. This is to avoid cross-contamination of additives between tubes and ensure accuracy of results.

- Always label blood bottles immediately after the samples are taken at the bedside next to the patient.

- Always follow trust policy and guidelines (especially for group and save samples as protocol varies between trusts).

Blood Cultures

Candidate's Instructions

You are the foundation year doctor on a medical ward. You have been informed by the nursing staff that a patient has spiked a temperature of 38.1°C. You decide to take blood cultures as part of the septic screen.

Demonstrate how you would do so using the equipment provided.

Examiner's Instructions

The candidate is a foundation year doctor on a medical ward. They have been asked to take blood cultures from a patient who has just spiked a temperature of 38.1°C.

The candidate will perform this skill on the dummy arm using the equipment provided. The actor will provide the voice of the patient.

Actor's Instructions

You are a patient on one of the medical wards. You have just spiked a temperature of 38.1°C. The candidate is a foundation doctor who has been called to take blood cultures.

You have had bloods taken before, and are happy to have these samples taken. You do not have any concerns about the procedure.

Blood Cultures

Task:	Achieved:	Not achieved:
Washes hands		
Introduces self		
Confirms patient name, DOB and hospital number		
Gains consent to take blood cultures		
Positions patient with forearm resting on cushion		
Selects the correct blood culture bottles and equipment, including sharps bin		
Removes tops from both blood culture bottles and cleans each with a separate alcohol wipe, and allows to dry.		
Applies tourniquet		
Selects appropriate vein		
Puts on gloves		
Cleans the area thoroughly with an alcohol wipe/ Chloroprep™		
Attaches needle to Vacutainer® correctly		
Warns patient to expect 'sharp scratch' or similar		
Retracts skin distally to stabilise vein and inserts needle correctly using aseptic non-touch technique		
Attaches blood culture bottles in the correct order (aerobic first) and withdraws 8-10mls of blood under vacuum		
Releases tourniquet		
Removes needle and immediately disposes of it in the sharps bin		
Applies pressure to venepuncture site and thanks patient		
Labels containers correctly by hand (or explains how to do so) and fills in the appropriate form		
Examiner's Global Mark	/5	
Actor / Helper's Global Mark	/5	
Total Station Mark	/30	

Learning points

- Blood cultures provide valuable information about the aetiology of an infection and help guide management. They should be taken as soon as bacteraemia is suspected, ideally before antibiotic therapy has been commenced

- It is important to maintain an Aseptic Non-Touch Technique (ANTT) whilst obtaining the blood sample as contamination can cause confusion and may lead to unnecessary investigations.

- It is important that blood cultures are filled appropriately. The minimum sample required is 8-10mls of blood. This helps to improve the diagnostic yield of the sample.

Death Verification and Certification

Candidate's Instructions

You are the foundation year doctor on call for the medical wards this evening. You have been called by the sister on the stroke ward and asked to attend to confirm the death of a patient. No resuscitation attempts have taken place as the patient has a valid do not attempt resuscitation form at the beginning of his notes.

Please demonstrate on the model the procedure you would carry to confirm death. Describe your actions to the examiner as you proceed.

Following this you will be asked to review a summary of the patients' notes and answer some questions.

Examiner's Instructions

This station contains two parts. Initially the student will need to verify death and demonstrate this on the model in the station. The patient who has died is an elderly gentleman with vascular dementia who has suffered a large disabling stroke. He has not made a good recovery and after consultation with his family has been commenced on end of life care. His death is expected and he has a valid DNACPR in place.

Please prompt the candidate if they do not mention documentation, ask them where they would write what has happened and what they would write.

At the 4 minute mark please present the student with the notes summary card in the station. Give them 1 minute to read this and then ask them the questions in the mark scheme regarding certification and the coroner.

Please ask them;
  What might be put in part 1a?
  What might be put in part 1b?
  What might be put in part 1c?
  What might be put in part 2?
  Whether this case requires referral to the coroner?
  To list at least 3 reasons for referring a patient death to the coroner

Actor's Instructions

You are the sister in charge on the Stroke unit. You were supervising this evening when a health care assistant asked you to check on Bernard as she thought he did not look right.

Bernard is an elderly gentleman with multi-infarct dementia, who was admitted with a large middle cerebral artery infarction. He did not improve with treatment, so after discussion with his family he was commenced on end of life care. He was being nursed in a side room and his death was expected. He had a valid DNACPR in place. In view of this you did not start CPR but have instead gathered his notes and asked the foundation doctor to verify his death. The family have been informed, but are not present.

You have the DNAR in your pile of notes as well as a notes summary which you will later give to the candidate.

Resource
Notes summation:

Bernard was a 85 year old retired civil servant. Two years ago he was diagnosed with multi-infarct dementia. He had hypertension and diabetes for the last 15 years. One evening his wife found him collapsed on the floor unable to move his right side. He was brought into hospital and admitted under your team with a diagnosis of stroke.

Despite the efforts of your team he died 6 days later. You had been present on the ward round the day before his death and discussed with the consultant the fact his GCS was declining. A DNACPR had been put in place in view of the severity of the neurological damage from the stroke and likely poor outcomes of CPR.

Death Verification and Certification

Task	Achieved	Not Achieved
Washes hands		
Introduces self to nurse and elicits appropriate details (time of death, persons present, expected death, valid DNACPR)		
Reviews patient's notes		
Confirms patient's identity with wrist band		
Observes patient for signs of life		
Observes for respiratory effort		
Checks response to verbal and tactile stimuli		
Palpates major pulse (carotid or femoral)		
Auscultates for heart sounds- for at least 1 minute		
Auscultates for breath sounds- for at least 2 minutes		
Inspects eyes and tests pupillary response to light		
Checks for a pacemaker		
Washes hands		
Documents findings in the patient's notes		
At this point please as the candidate to read the summary and then ask them if they were filling out the death certificate, for cause of death:		
What may be put in 1(a)? Cerebrovascular accident		
What may be put in 1(b)? Atherosclerosis		
What may be put in 1(c)? Hypertension		
What may be put in 2? Diabetes Mellitus, Multi-infarct dementia		
Would this death need to be reported to the coroner? **No**		
What are the reasons for referring a patient to the coroner? (if candidate can give 3 award mark)		
Examiner's Global Mark	/5	
Actor / Helper's Global Mark	/5	
Total Station Mark	/30	

Learning Points

- It is important to verify whether the death is expected, whether there is a valid DNACPR in place and the patient's identity.

- If there are absent respiratory movements, the patient is unresponsive, there are no pulses, no heart sounds, no breath sounds, pupils are fixed and dilated you can verify death.

- Reasons for referral to coroner are as follows;
  - Death was violent/ unnatural/ suspicious
  - Death may be due to an accident
  - Death may be due to suicide
  - Death in custody
  - Death may be due to an industrial disease or as a result of employment
  - Death occurred during an operation or before recovery from an anaesthetic
  - Death within 24 hours of hospital admission
  - Cause of death unknown or in doubt

History Taking

Chest Pain

Candidate's Instructions

You are the foundation year doctor working on the acute medical take. Molly is a 57 year old lady who has presented with chest pain. Please take a focused history from her.

At 6 minutes you will be asked to present your history, give a differential diagnosis and provide a management plan.

Examiner's Instructions

The candidate has been asked to take a focused history from a patient. Molly is a 57-year-old librarian. She has been experiencing intermittent chest pain whilst walking the dog after work. This has been going on for the past few weeks. GTN has helped with the pain. Whilst out shopping with her daughter today she developed tight, central chest pain associated with nausea and breathlessness that lasted over an hour. GTN spray did not relieve the pain.

The patient is able to lie flat at night without breathlessness. She has no ankle swelling. She has a PMHx of type 2 diabetes (diet controlled), high blood pressure, high cholesterol and angina.

The patient's father died of an MI at the age of 62. There are no other medical problems in the patient's family.

The patient takes aspirin, losartan, atorvastatin and GTN spray. She has no drug allergies.

The patient smoke has smoked 20 cigarettes a day for the past 20 years, but has recently cut down to 10 a day. She drinks a glass of wine an evening. She lives with her husband and 18-year-old daughter.

The patient is worried that she is having a heart attack, especially as her father dies at a similar age.

At 6 minutes please stop the candidate ask them to present their findings and suggest a management plan.

Actor's Instructions

You are a 57 year old librarian. You have been experiencing intermittent central chest pain lasting only a few minutes for the last few weeks whilst walking the dog after work. Using your GTN spray has helped to ease the pain. Whilst out shopping in town today with your daughter, the chest pain came on but this time it lasted over an hour. It was a tight sensation in the middle of your chest and you began to feel very breathless and nauseous. GTN spray did not relieve the pain this time. You have been able to lie flat at night without getting breathless and have not noticed any ankle swelling.

Your other medical problems include T2DM (diet controlled), high blood pressure, high cholesterol and angina.

Your father died of a heart attack aged 62 but there are no other medical problems in the family.

You take aspirin, losartan, atorvastatin and GTN spray. You have no drug allergies.

You have been smoking 30 cigarettes a day for around 20 years but did recently cut down to ten cigarettes a day. You drink a glass of wine every night.
You live with your husband and 18-year-old daughter.

You are very worried that you are having a heart attack and that you might die especially given that your father died of a heart attack at around your age.

Chest Pain

Task	Achieved	Not Achieved
Washes hands		
Introduces self		
Confirms patient details (name, age, occupation)		
Gains consent to take history		
Starts consultation with open question		
Establishes pain history (site, onset, character, radiation, exacerbating and reliving factors, timing)		
Enquires specifically about cardiovascular risk factors (smoking, family history, diet, exercise)		
Elicits systems review (dyspnoea, cough, sweating, nausea, vomiting, palpitations, syncope, oedema, PND, orthopnoea)		
Elicits past medical history		
Elicits family history		
Elicits drug history and drug allergies		
Elicits social history		
Elicits alcohol history		
Elicits smoking history		
Enquires about patient's ideas, concerns and expectations		
Summarises back to patient		
Shows empathy and avoids jargon		
Presents findings in clear, concise manner		
Gives sensible differential diagnosis (e.g. unstable angina, NSTEMI, STEMI)		
Gives sensible management plan (e.g. examination, observations, bloods including troponins, ECG, CXR etc.)		
Examiner's Global Mark	/5	
Actor / Helper's Global Mark	/5	
Total Station Mark	/30	

Learning Points

- Remember to explore the patients Ideas, Concerns and Expectations (ICE). By exploring these aspects of the history the patient may reveal more clinical details and allow you to focus your history further. Time invested here is time saved elsewhere.

- If you suspect ischaemic heart disease it is important to establish whether the patient has any cardiovascular risk factors (high cholesterol, smoking history, diabetes, hypertension, strong family history).

- Don't forget to include use of over the counter medications and drug allergies as an important component of your drug history.

Shortness of Breath

Candidate's Instructions

You are the foundation year doctor working on the acute medical take. Frank is a 75 year old man who has presented with shortness of breath. Please take a focused history from her.

At 6 minutes you will be asked to present your history, give a differential diagnosis and provide a management plan.

Examiner's Instructions

The candidate has been asked to take a focused history from a patient.

The patient is a 75-year-old retired school teacher. Over the last few weeks he has become increasingly short of breath on exertion. He is only able to move between rooms at home before becoming breathless. 6 months ago he was able to walk to the local shops. He does not feel breathless at rest. Sleeping has become increasingly difficult as he becomes breathless when lying down flat. He wakes up a few times a night gasping for breath. He has now resorted to sleeping in an armchair. His ankles have become swollen over the past few weeks. He has no wheeze, chest pain, cough, fever, palpitations or weight loss. He has no recent ravel history.

His mother had a heart attack in her 60s and his father died of lung cancer aged 82.

He had a large heart attack 6 months ago and required 2 stents. He also has hypertension, and high cholesterol.

His medications include aspirin, clopidogrel, atorvastatin, ramipril, bisoprolol, lansoprazole and GTN. He has a penicillin allergy (rash).

He is an ex-smoker. He smoked 15 a day for 20 years but gave up aged 40. He drinks two glasses of wine a week.

He lives in a house with stairs and is the main carer for his wife who has Alzhiemer's. He does not want to be admitted to hospital as he's concerned about how his wife will manage.

At 6 minutes please stop the candidate ask them to present their findings and suggest a management plan.

Actor's Instructions

You are a 75 year old retired school teacher. Over the last few weeks you have become increasingly short of breath particularly on doing any form of activity. You are only able to walk to the bathroom before getting short of breath. Six months ago you were able to the shops down the road without much difficulty. You do not feel breathless when resting. However sleeping has become increasingly difficult as you become very breathless when lying flat and wake up at least a few times a night gasping for breath. You have resorted to sleeping in your arm chair. On direct questioning you note that your ankles have become increasingly swollen over the last few weeks. You deny wheeze, chest pain, cough, fever, palpitations and weight loss. You have not travelled recently.

Your mother had a heart attack in her 60s. Your father died of lung cancer aged 82.

You had a large heart attack six months ago and required 2 stents. You have high blood pressure and high cholesterol.

You take aspirin, clopidogrel, atorvastatin, ramipril, bisoprolol, lansoprazole and GTN spray. You are allergic to penicillin and have previously developed a rash when taking it.

You smoked 15 a day for 20 years but gave up at the age of 40. You drink two glasses of wine/week.

You live in a house with stairs with your wife who has Alzheimer's dementia. You are her full time carer. You are adamant that you cannot be admitted to hospital as your wife struggled to cope when you were admitted six months ago.

Shortness of Breath

Task	Achieved	Not Achieved
Washes hands		
Introduces self		
Confirms patient details (name, age, occupation)		
Gains consent to take history		
Starts consultation with open question		
Takes focussed dyspnoea history (onset, duration, severity, timing, precipitating factors, relieving factors)		
Enquires about exercise tolerance		
Elicits systems review (cough, chest pain, sweating, nausea, vomiting, palpitations, syncope, oedema, PND, orthopnoea)		
Elicits past medical history		
Elicits family history		
Elicits drug history and drug allergies		
Elicits social history		
Elicits alcohol history		
Elicits smoking history		
Enquires about patient's ideas, concerns and expectations		
Summarises back to patient		
Shows empathy and avoids jargon		
Presents findings in clear, concise manner		
Gives sensible differential diagnosis (e.g. heart failure, COPD, pulmonary fibrosis)		
Gives sensible management plan (e.g. examination, observations, bloods including BNP, ECG, CXR etc.)		
Examiner's Global Mark	/5	
Actor / Helper's Global Mark	/5	
Total Station Mark	/30	

Learning Points

- Remember that shortness of breath may be due to respiratory, cardiac or metabolic causes.

- Symptoms that are suggestive of heart failure include breathlessness on exertion, leg swelling, orthopnoea and paroxysmal nocturnal dyspnoea.

- The New York Heart Association classification can be used to quantify patient's symptoms

No limitation of physical activity
Slight limitation of activity, comfortable at rest.
Marked limitation of activity, comfortable at rest.
Symptoms of heart failure at rest

Abdominal Pain

Candidate's Instructions

You are the foundation year doctor working on the acute medical take. Matthew is a 48 year old investment banker who has presented with abdominal pain. Please take a focussed history from him.

At 6 minutes you will be asked to present your history, give a differential diagnosis and provide a management plan.

Examiner's Instructions

The candidate has been asked to take a focused history from a patient.

The patient is a 48 year old investment banker, who works in the city. He has been experiencing epigastric pain on and off for the past few weeks. Since yesterday it has become progressively worse. He normally experiences the pain in the evenings a few hours after eating, and occasionally at night. The pain is aggravated by alcohol intake and spicy foods. He feels nauseous but has never vomited. The patient has presented today following an episode of vomiting, in which he noted some black spots. His stools have been noticeably darker recently. He has not lost any weight or lost his appetite.

He had an appendicectomy aged 17, but is otherwise fit and well.

His mother died of bowel cancer, but there are no other medical problems in the family.

His work has been very stressful recently, and he has been skipping meals. He gets recurrent tension headaches for which he has been taking paracetamol and ibuprofen. He buys these medications over the counter. He has also been drinking more than usual around 26 units/week. He is an occasional social smoker. You live with 2 other work colleagues.

At 6 minutes please stop the candidate ask them to present their findings and suggest a management plan.

Actor's Instructions

You are a 48 year old investment banker working in the city. You have been experiencing epigastric pain for the last few weeks but since yesterday it has become considerably worse. You usually experience the pain in the evenings a few hours after eating and occasionally at night. The pain is aggravated by alcohol intake and spicy foods. Associated with the pain, you feel nauseous but have never vomited. The reason you have come to the hospital today is because in addition to the pain worsening in severity you have had an episode of vomiting this morning. You noticed black spots in the vomit. Your stool has been noticeably darker as well. You have not experienced any other symptoms including weight loss or reduced appetite.

You are normally fit and well although did have an open appendicectomy aged 17.

Your mother died of bowel cancer but there are no other medical problems in the family.

On direct questioning you reveal that work has been very stressful lately, you barely have time to get lunch most days. You recurrently get headaches and have been taking paracetemol and ibuprofen daily as a preventative measure. You buy this over the counter. You have no drug allergies. You also have been drinking much more than usual, around 26 units/week. You gave up smoking 5 years ago but do occasionally smoke at parties. You live with two other work colleagues. You are worried you will need surgery for whatever is going on and you are adamant that you cannot have surgery no matter what.

Abdominal Pain

Task	Achieved	Not Achieved
Washes hands		
Introduces self		
Confirms patient details (name, age, occupation)		
Gains consent to take history		
Starts consultation with open question		
Establishes pain history including duration, onset, timing, exacerbating and relieving factors		
Elicits additional symptoms (dysphagia, weight loss, appetite, nausea, vomiting, altered bowel habit, jaundice and fever)		
Elicits systems review (cough, chest pain, sweating, nausea, vomiting, palpitations, syncope, oedema, PND, orthopnoea)		
Enquires specifically about peptic ulcer disease, GORD and liver disease		
Elicits past medical and surgical history		
Elicits drug history and drug allergies (specifically asks about NSAIDs, steroids, anticoagulants)		
Elicits social history		
Elicits alcohol history		
Elicits smoking history		
Enquires about patient's ideas, concerns and expectations		
Summarises back to patient		
Shows empathy and avoids jargon		
Presents findings in clear, concise manner		
Gives sensible differential diagnosis (e.g. gastritis, peptic ulcer disease, GORD)		
Gives sensible management plan (e.g. examination, observations, bloods including FBC, Coag, Amylase, X-match, ECG, erect CXR etc.)		
Examiner's Global Mark	/5	
Actor / Helper's Global Mark	/5	
Total Station Mark	/30	

Learning Points

- It is really important to enquire about NSAID use if you are concerned about gastrointestinal bleeding. These often aren't prescribed and patient's buy them over the counter, therefore may not volunteer them as part of their drug history.

- It is important to try and quantify somebody's alcohol intake as much as possible. Sometimes patient can be vague when describing their alcohol consumption. Men and women are now both advised not to drink more than 14 units a week on a regular basis and to spread their drinking over three or more days if they regularly drink as much as 14 units a week

- As a rough guide:
    - A small glass (175ml) of white wine is approximately 2 units
    - A pint of low strength lager or beer is 2 units
    - A pint of high strength lager or beer is 3 units
    - A single shot of spirits is 1 unit

Diarrhoea

Candidate's instructions

You are a foundation doctor on attachment to a general practice surgery. A 23-year-old man has come to his GP with a history of diarrhoea. He is normally well with no other medical conditions. Please take a focussed history from him.

At 6 minutes you will be asked to present your history, give a differential diagnosis and provide a management plan.

Examiner's instructions

The candidate has been asked to take a focused history from a patient.

The patient is a 23-year-old man has come to his GP with a history of diarrhoea. He is normally well with no other medical conditions. His symptoms started 4 weeks ago. Initially the patient thought he had food poisoning following a recent holiday to Spain. The patient is opening his bowels 5-6 times per day, and it is often bloody. He often experiences abdominal pain that is worse before he opens his bowels. He has symptoms of urgency, and has had some faecal incontinence. He has lots 3-4kg in weight and is fatigued. He has no history of mouth ulcers, eye or joint pain or rashes.

He has no other medical conditions and does not take any regular medications. He drinks alcohol occasionally, but started smoking a couple of years ago.

He has a family history of type 2-diabetes and his Grandma recently had a stroke. There is no family history of cancer.

He is embarrassed about coming to see the GP and his symptoms are starting to impact on his social life. He works as a bus driver and has had to take time off because of his symptoms.

At 6 minutes please stop the candidate ask them to present their findings and suggest a management plan.

Actor's instructions

You are a 23-year-old man who has gone to your GP because of bloody diarrhoea. This started around 4 weeks ago. Initially you thought it was food poisoning from a recent holiday to Spain, but it hasn't gone away. You open your bowels between 5-6 times a day and it is often bloody. You often experience severe abdominal pain that is worse before you open your bowels. You often having urgency and on one occasion have not made it to the toilet. You have noticed around 3-4 kg weight loss since this started. You haven't had any mouth ulcers, eye or joint pain or rashes but are often tired.

You are normally well with other medical conditions and don't take any regular medications. You don't drink much but started smoking a few years ago. You have a family history of diabetes (type 2) and your grandma recently had a stroke. There is no family history of cancer.

You were reluctant to come to your GP and are very embarrassed about the diarrhoea. Since not making it to the toilet you have been worried about going out with friends, which has affected your social life. You work as a bus driver and have had to take time off work.

Diarrhoea

Task	Achieved	Not Achieved
Washes hands		
Introduces self		
Confirms patient details (name, age, occupation)		
Gains consent to take history		
Starts consultation with open question		
Establishes diarrhoea history (onset, frequency, pain, night-time symptoms, presence of blood, consistency, mucus, tenesmus)		
Elicits important additional symptoms (weight loss, fever, malaise, rashes, eye symptoms, appetite, nausea, vomiting)		
Asks about travel history and ill contacts		
Elicits systems review		
Elicits past medical and surgical history		
Elicits drug history and drug allergies (specifically asks about NSAIDs, steroids, anticoagulants)		
Elicits social history		
Elicits alcohol history		
Elicits smoking history		
Enquires about patient's ideas, concerns and expectations		
Summarises back to patient		
Shows empathy and avoids jargon		
Presents findings in clear, concise manner		
Gives sensible differential diagnosis (e.g. infective diarrhoea, inflammatory bowel disease)		
Gives sensible management plan (e.g. examination, observations, bloods including FBC, CRP, ESR, stool cultures, AXR etc.)		
Examiner's Global Mark	/5	
Actor / Helper's Global Mark	/5	
Total Station Mark	/30	

Learning points

- It is essential to ask about foreign travel and unwell contacts. The majority of diarrhoea in young adults is infectious.

- It is important to ask patients' the impact their condition is having on their job and social life. Listen to the patient and pick up on their non-verbal cues. Diarrhoea is affecting this patient's work and social life. It is important to pick up on this.

- Diarrhoea red flags include weight loss, bleeding, night-time symptoms, family history of bowel cancer, abdominal masses and anaemia.

Collapse

Candidate's Instructions

You are a foundation year doctor in the emergency department. Brenda is a 71-year-old lady who has presented to the emergency department with collapse. Please take a focussed history.

At 6 minutes you will be asked to present your history, give a differential diagnosis and provide a management plan.

Examiner's Instructions

The candidate has been asked to take focussed history from a patient. The patient is a 71-year-old lady called Brenda who has presented to the emergency department with collapse.

Prior to the event the patient was sat watching TV. On standing she felt nauseous and light headed. Her husband noted that she was pale. The patient did not experience any chest pain, breathlessness or palpitations.

The next thing the patient remembers is being on the floor. Her husband says she was only unconscious for a few seconds. There was no incontinence, tongue biting or seizure activity noted. She did not sustain any injuries.

She was disorientated and confused for a few seconds only. She made a quick recovery. Her husband was concerned so he bought her to the emergency department.

She has no history of syncope, but over the past few weeks has been feeling dizzy especially when changing position. Last week the patient felt dizzy whilst gardening, but her symptoms resolved after lying down. She has been well otherwise, but admits to not drinking enough fluids.

She has a history of high blood pressure, but this is now well controlled with medications. She used to be on a blood pressure medication that made her ankles swell, but this has recently been changed to bendroflumethiazide.

The correct diagnosis is syncope due to postural hypotension (secondary to dehydration and antihypertensives/diuretics).

At 6 minutes please stop the candidate ask them to present their findings and suggest a management plan.

Actor's Instructions

You are a 71-year-old lady who has presented to the emergency department with collapse.

Before the event: You were sat watching TV and went to make a cup of tea. When you stood up you felt nauseous and light-headed. Your husband said you went as pale as a ghost. You did not have any chest pain, breathlessness or palpitations.

During: The next thing you remember is being on the floor in the middle of the living room. Your husband said you were only unconscious for a few seconds. You did not have any incontinence and did not bite your tongue or have any jerking movement of your limbs during this episode. You did not have any injury during the fall.

After: You felt a bit disorientated and confused for a few seconds but after that you felt ok. You feel well now. Your husband was concerned and made you come to the ED.

You have never collapsed before, although over the last few weeks you have had some dizziness. This dizziness occurs first thing in the morning when you get out of bed or when you stand up from a chair. In fact, last week you felt dizzy when doing the gardening and had to have a lie down. You just thought it was due to the hot weather and your age. You have been well in yourself otherwise with no other symptoms and no recent illness. If asked you don't drink much water because you don't really like the taste but you do drink a few cups of tea a day, which perhaps isn't enough during the summer.

PMH: You have very little past medical history apart from the fact that your blood pressure used to be high. However, this is now well controlled because they have recently increased your medication.

Medication: You were taking a pill for your blood pressure, but it made your ankles swollen which didn't look very nice in the summer when wearing a skirt. So about a month ago your lovely GP started you on a new tablet and you take one in the morning. You can't remember what it is called but you've got the packet with you: 'bendroflumethiazide 2.5mg'

Collapse

Task	Achieved	Not Achieved
Washes hands		
Introduces self		
Confirms patient details (name, age, occupation)		
Gains consent to take history		
Starts consultation with open question		
Establishes details prior to collapse (preceding symptoms, posture, prodrome, provoking factors)		
Elicits details during the collapse (duration, LOC, jerky movements, incontinence)		
Elicits details of behaviour after collapse (confusion/injuries/altered mental state)		
Elicits systems review		
Elicits past medical and surgical history		
Elicits drug history and drug allergies (specifically asks about anti-hypertensives, diuretics)		
Elicits social history		
Elicits alcohol history		
Elicits smoking history		
Enquires about patient's ideas, concerns and expectations		
Summarises back to patient		
Shows empathy and avoids jargon		
Presents findings in clear, concise manner		
Gives sensible differential diagnosis (e.g. postural hypotension, vasovagal syncope, carotid sinus hypersensitivity,cardiogenic)		
Gives sensible management plan (e.g. examination, observations, bloods, L/S BP, medication review, ECG)		
Examiner's Global Mark	/5	
Actor / Helper's Global Mark	/5	
Total Station Mark	/30	

Learning Points

- When taking a syncope history think about the **3P's**;
    Posture
    Prodrome
    Provoking Factors

- An eyewitness account may be crucial in determining whether an event was a transient loss of consciousness or seizure

- TIA's do not cause loss of consciousness, and should not form part of the differential here.

Weight loss

Candidate's Instructions

You are a foundation year doctor attached to a general medical ward. Brenda is a 65-year old lady who has presented with weight loss. Please take a focussed history.

At 6 minutes you will be asked to present your history, give a differential diagnosis and provide a management plan.

Examiner's Instructions

The candidate has been asked to take focussed history from a patient.

The patient is a 65-year-old lady who has presented to the GP with weight loss. She has been losing weight for the past 6 months, but has not been trying to lose weight. She has noticed that her clothes are loose. She has had some diarrhoea; prior to this she had a normal bowel habit. She has noticed that her appetite has reduced, and she often skips meals. She is also a bit irritable, and has been feeling tremulous and experiencing palpitations intermittently.

She has no past medical history and does not take any regular medications. Her brother and sister are diabetic.

She is concerned as her mother died of breast cancer in her 60s, and lost weight in her terminal phase. She is concerned that she may have cancer.

At 6 minutes please stop the candidate ask them to present their findings and suggest a management plan.

Actor's Instructions

You have had a nine-month history of weight loss and are starting to get concerned as you have not been trying to lose weight. You have noticed that your clothes are loose. You have had some loose stool for six months with occasional periods of constipation in between. Prior to this, your bowel motions were regular. You have also noticed that you are eating less and sometimes you might skip lunch as you don't feel hungry. You have noticed that you can be irritable at times and have had intermittent palpitations.

You have no other medical conditions. Your brother and sister are diabetic.

You have no allergies and do not take any regular medications.

You have been feeling worried because your mother died of breast cancer in her 60s and she lost a lot of weight in her terminal phase. You have decided to come in to find out what the cause of your weight loss might be, and whether you also have cancer.

Weight loss

Task	Achieved	Not Achieved
Washes hands		
Introduces self		
Confirms patient details (name, age, occupation)		
Gains consent to take history		
Starts consultation with open question		
Establishes details of weight loss (duration, amount, loss of appetite, dietary intake)		
Screens for malignancy (dysphagia, abdominal distension, change in bowel habit, blood in stools)		
Elicits systems review in particular considers diabetes, hyperthyroidism, mood disorders,		
Elicits past medical and surgical history		
Elicits drug history and drug allergies (specifically asks about anti-hypertensives, diuretics)		
Elicits social history		
Elicits alcohol history		
Elicits smoking history		
Elicits family history in particular relating to cancer		
Enquires about patient's ideas, concerns and expectations		
Summarises back to patient		
Shows empathy and avoids jargon		
Presents findings in clear, concise manner		
Gives sensible differential diagnosis (e.g. malignancy, hyperthyroidism, malabsorption)		
Gives sensible management plan (e.g. examination, observations, bloods including coeliac screen, thyroid function, FBC, medication review, 2 week wait colonoscopy)		
Examiner's Global Mark	/5	
Actor / Helper's Global Mark	/5	
Total Station Mark	/30	

Learning Points

- This is a difficult case. The differential diagnosis of weight loss is wide-ranging including endocrine disorders, malignancy, chronic disease, malabsorption, poor dentition, alcohol excess and depression.

- Try to have a 'surgical sieve' as a template to use to create a list of differential diagnoses in your mind when taking a history. This will help guide your structure and questions you ask.

- Red flags for weight loss include respiratory symptoms, bony pain, "B" symptoms, iron deficiency anaemia, increasing age amongst others.

Red Hot Joint

Candidate's instructions

You are the foundation year doctor in the emergency department. A 32-year-old lady has attended complaining of pain and swelling in her right wrist. She is haemodynamically stable, but has a temperature of 38.7 °C. Please take a focussed history.

At 6 minutes you will be asked to present your history, give a differential diagnosis and provide a management plan.

Examiner's instructions

The candidate has been asked to take focussed history from a patient.

The patient is a 32-year-old lady who has presented to the emergency department complaining of pain and swelling in her right wrist. She is haemodynamically stable but she has a temperature of 38.7 degrees and is clearly in pain.

The patient has had pain and swelling in the wrist for 2 days. She has been taking regular paracetamol and ibuprofen, with no relief. She has felt generally unwell and feverish. Prior to this episode the patient was well and has not had any bowel or bladder symptoms. She has not had any surgery or sustained any trauma to the wrist.

She has a past medical history of Rheumatoid arthritis, but this normally affects the small joints of her hands and feet. She takes methotrexate. She has a penicillin allergy that causes anaphylaxis. There is a history of diabetes in the family. She works in finance but has had to take time off work. She is in a stable relationship and has not had any new sexual partners. She smokes 10 cigarettes a day, but does not drink any alcohol.

At 6 minutes please stop the candidate ask them to present their findings and suggest a management plan.

Actor's instructions

You are a 32-year-old lady presenting to the emergency department with pain and swelling in your right wrist.

Your wrist has been increasingly painful, red and swollen for 2 days and you are now finding you cannot move the joint due to a severe 'burning' pain in it. You have been taking regular paracetamol and ibuprofen, but it hasn't helped. You have felt generally unwell and feverish at home but have not measured your temperature. Prior to this episode you have been well and you have no bowel or bladder symptoms. You have not had any recent surgery or injuries to your wrist.

You have a background of rheumatoid arthritis, which is difficult to control and normally affects the small joint of both your hand and wrists. For this you take methotrexate. You have an allergy to penicillin (anaphylaxis). Diabetes runs in your family, but you are not diabetic.

You work in finance, but have been unable to go to the office with this pain. You are in a stable relationship and have not had any new sexual partners. You are a vegetarian, smoke 10 cigarettes a day and do not drink alcohol.

You become quite tearful during the consultation because you are in pain and you are worried because this is not like your normal pain.

Red hot swollen joint

Task	Achieved	Not Achieved
Washes hands		
Introduces self		
Confirms patient details (name, age, occupation)		
Gains consent to take history		
Starts consultation with open question		
Elicits appropriate pain history		
Screens for causes of a red hot swollen joint (crystal arthropathies, inflammatory joint disease, post-surgical, trauma)		
Takes brief sexual history		
Elicits past medical and surgical history		
Elicits drug history and drug allergies		
Elicits social history		
Elicits alcohol history		
Elicits smoking history		
Elicits family history		
Enquires about patient's ideas, concerns and expectations		
Summarises back to patient		
Shows empathy and avoids jargon		
Presents findings in clear, concise manner		
Gives sensible differential diagnosis (e.g. septic arthritis, rheumatoid arthritis)		
Gives sensible management plan (e.g. examination, observations, bloods including FBC, CRP, ESR, x-ray, joint aspirate)		
Examiner's Global Mark	/5	
Actor / Helper's Global Mark	/5	
Total Station Mark	/30	

Learning points

- Septic arthritis is an important differential for a red hot swollen joint. Always ask about risk factors for septic arthritis when taking a history for this presentation:

    Any damage to the joint (e.g. arthritis, gout or previous injury)

    Immunosuppression (e.g from medication or diseases like HIV)

    Diabetes

    Any surgery to the joint or prosthetic joints

- It is important to take a sexual history from any patient presenting with a red hot swollen joint and consider the diagnosis of reactive arthritis.

- Screening for extra-articular symptoms and systemic symptoms may help you to narrow your diagnosis.

Collateral History

Candidate's Instructions

You are the foundation year doctor on the medical take. An 83-year-old lady has been brought into the acute medical unit. The patient is confused and unable to give a history, but the patient's next of kin is present and willing to give a collateral history. Please take a focussed collateral history.

At 6 minutes you will be asked to present your history, give a differential diagnosis and provide a management plan.

Examiner's Instructions

The candidate has been asked to take focussed collateral history from a relative.

The relative is the patient's daughter. She has bought her mother to hospital because she has been generally unwell for the past 3 days. Her mother has had a chesty cough for the past 2 weeks, and has complained of feeling hot and cold. Her mother is usually incontinent of urine, but manages her pads herself. Over the past 2 days she has smelt strongly of urine. The patient's mother has taken to her bed over the past 3 days due to illness.

Her mother is occasionally forgetful, and is usually orientated to time, place and person. Her mother has no formal diagnosis of dementia. Her mother has been increasingly confused and hallucinating over the past 2 days. This is not normal for her. She is not aware of any other symptoms, falls or head injury.

Her mother has a history of hypertension, high cholesterol and heart trouble following a heart attack many years ago. Her mother takes bisoprolol, ramipril, spironolactone, aspirin and simvastatin. Her medications are in a dosette box and she is compliant with her medications.

Her mother lives alone in a bungalow. She has no formal package of care, but her daughter visits every other day. Her mother is usually independent with her ADLs and walks with a stick. She attends a social club once a week. She does not drink alcohol and has never smoked.

Her daughter is concerned about her mother's current confusion and wants to know if it will get better. She does not think she will cope alone at home in her current state.

At 6 minutes please stop the candidate ask them to present their findings and suggest a management plan.

Actor's Instructions

Your 83-year-old mother has been admitted to the acute medical unit after a few days of feeling generally unwell. You are happy to give a collateral history as you are the patient's next of kin and you brought her to hospital.

You are initially quite vague about symptoms, but every day you visited your mother the last 3 days, she kept saying "I don't feel very well" or "I feel under the weather". When asked specifically, you're not sure if your mother had a fever as you did not measure her temperature, but she did complain of feeling hot and cold last night; she had a chesty sounding cough for the last week, she did not show you any phlegm brought up, she is normally incontinent of urine (stress incontinence) but changes pads herself so you cannot comment on any urinary symptoms; however, you have noticed she smells quite strongly of urine the last 2 days. She has been bedbound for the last 3 days with this illness.

When asked about your mother's baseline cognitive function, you say she is becoming quite "senile", slightly more forgetful the last year or so since her husband died, but she has no formal diagnosis of dementia. She is normally fully orientated to where she is and the time of day and recognizes people well – she only occasionally misplaces things around the house e.g. keys. When asked specifically, she is definitely more confused very suddenly the last 2 days than what is normal for her. Her level of confusion keeps has kept fluctuating over these 2 days. Yesterday, she did not recognize you and even mentioned seeing elephants coming out of from under her bed, when there was nothing there! She has never had hallucinations in the past. You are not aware of any other symptoms. She has not sustained any head injury.

Your mother has high blood pressure, high cholesterol and "heart trouble"since a heart attack 10 years ago. She is on bisoprolol, ramipril, spironolactone, aspirin and simvastatin. She uses a dosette box and is always compliant with her medicines. You think the dose of ramipril may have been increased recently. She has no allergies. She lives alone in a bungalow with no package of care, but you live nearby and visit for an hour every other day. She is normally independent, mobilising with a walking stick. She goes to an Age Concern social club once a week. She does not drink alcohol and has never smoked.

If asked directly, your main concern is whether your mother's confusion will get better. You are worried that she would not be able to cope alone at home in her new current state.

Collateral History

Task	Achieved	Not Achieved
Washes hands		
Introduces self		
Confirms patient details (name, age, occupation)		
Clarifies who they are speaking to and relationship to patient and gains consent to take collateral history		
Starts consultation with open question		
Elicits history of confusion (timing, onset, features, course i.e. fluctuating, progressive)		
Elicits physical/ infective symptoms		
Elicits baseline cognitive status		
Elicits past medical and surgical history		
Elicits drug history (including medication changes and compliance) and drug allergies		
Elicits social history (enquires about baseline function)		
Elicits alcohol history		
Elicits smoking history		
Elicits family history		
Enquires about patient's ideas, concerns and expectations		
Summarises back to patient		
Shows empathy and avoids jargon		
Presents findings in clear, concise manner		
Gives sensible differential diagnosis (e.g. acute delirium, chest infection, pneumonia, urinary tract infection)		
Gives sensible management plan (e.g. examination, observations, bloods including FBC, CRP, U&E, LFTs, TFTs, B12, Folate, Ferritin etc.)		
Examiner's Global Mark	/5	
Actor / Helper's Global Mark	/5	
Total Station Mark	/30	

Learning Points

- The key in this case is determining whether the onset of confusion was acute, chronic or acute-on-chronic. Never make assumptions that an elderly patient's confusion is due to dementia without getting a collateral history of their baseline cognition.

- The social history is crucial, particularly in finding out how independent or dependent a patient normally is with activities of daily living and mobility. This information is best gathered from someone close to the patient, who sees them regularly and can gauge a decline in their health. It will help with discharge planning as you determine whether the patient would be safe at home.

- Alongside the collateral history, confused patients will need full examination, a formal bedside cognitive assessment (e.g. AMTS) and a confusion screen as below. Don't forget to mention these to the examiner at the end of the station:

  - Bloods – FBC, U&Es, LFTs, CRP, TFTs, B12, folate
  - Urine dip +/- MCS
  - ECG
  - Chest x-ray
  - (CT head)

Communication/ Ethics

Breaking Bad News

Candidate's Instructions

You are the foundation year doctor on a geriatric ward and over the last 48 hours one of your patients has deteriorated and is approaching end of life. Your consultant has asked you to inform the family who are waiting in the relative's room.

Patient details

Humphrey, aged 86, has been in hospital for 3 days being treated for pneumonia. This is his 5th admission with aspiration pneumonia this year. Despite IV antibiotics and high flow oxygen he is failing to improve and respond to treatment. His oxygen saturations are 84% on 15L via a non-rebreathe mask, his blood pressure is low, he is starting to become oedematous with fluids and his urine output is poor. At the time of admission a DNACPR was discussed with his family, and a ceiling of ward-based treatment agreed.

Examiner's Instructions

This is a communication station. The candidate has been asked to inform a family that their relative is deteriorating and approaching end of life. Please assess their communication skills.

Patient details

Humphrey, aged 86, has been in hospital for 3 days being treated for pneumonia. This is his 5th admission with aspiration pneumonia this year. At the time of admission a DNACPR was discussed with his family, and a ceiling of ward-based treatment agreed. Despite IV antibiotics and high flow oxygen he is failing to improve and respond to treatment. His oxygen saturations are 84% on 15L via a non-rebreathe mask, his blood pressure is low, he is starting to become oedematous with fluids and his urine output is poor. A decision has been made to stop active treatment.

Actor's Instructions

You are Humphrey's wife. You have been happily married for 50 years. Humphrey has been very unwell over the last 2 years and has had a poor quality of life in a nursing home. He has been in hospital for the last 3 days being treated for pneumonia. You were asked to come into hospital this morning because the nurse said he wasn't very well overnight. You are waiting in the relatives' room to speak to a doctor and get an update on his condition.

You are expecting him to recover from this illness but you wouldn't want his quality of life to be any worse, and neither would he. He has been unwell in hospital before and he has always made a recovery. Your outlook is positive and you think that he'll be ok in a few days. A DNACPR was discussed with you at the start of Humphrey's admission, and you were in agreement with this.

A small part of you is worried that he might not make it through this illness, if this was the case you would be devastated but you understand that this would be better than him suffering a worse quality of life. You would want him to have a peaceful pain free death and he would want his family around him.

Breaking Bad News

Task:	Achieved	Not Achieved
Introduces self		
Confirms name and relationship to patient		
Asks if relative would like anyone else to be present		
Explores relatives understanding of events to date		
Clarifies and recaps on these events		
Asks relative how much they would like to know		
Gives a warning shot		
Explains clinical situation		
Doesn't give false hope, makes relative aware that patient is approaching end of life		
Explains use of palliative care drugs		
Asks about religious beliefs, offers chaplaincy		
Asks about preferred place of care		
Explains support available e.g. palliative care team, specialist nurses		
Tells relative what to expect next		
Invites questions		
Summarise		
Information given in a truthful and sensitive manner		
Acknowledges emotion and responds with empathy		
Gives sufficient pauses/allows silence		
Clarifies patient understanding throughout		
Avoids medical jargon		
Examiner's Global Mark	/5	
Actor / Helper's Global Mark	/5	
Total Station Mark	/30	

Learning Points

- Always start with an open question and clarify what the relative knows already and what they would like to know. This will help you to start this conversation at a place of mutual understanding.

- It is important to reiterate that palliative care medication will not speed up death, but aims to alleviate symptoms that could cause distress.

- Palliative care focuses on improving quality of life and it takes into account physical, spiritual, psychological and social needs of the patient and family. Try to address these four topics when discussing end of life care.

Explanation Type 2 Diabetes

Candidate's Instructions

You are a foundation year doctor attached to a General Practice. Edward is a 43-year-old gentleman who has recently had some routine blood tests. These blood tests show that he has Type 2 Diabetes. The diabetic nurse at the practice has asked you to inform the patient of his diagnosis and explain the condition.

Examiner's Instructions

This is a communication station. The candidate has been asked to explain a diagnosis of Type-2 Diabetes to a patient. Please assess their communication skills.

The patient is a 43-year-old lorry driver, who has been called back to the surgery following some recent blood tests. He is unaware that these blood tests show that he has Type 2 Diabetes. He is overweight and has hypertension and high cholesterol. He is a smoker of 20 cigarettes per day.

His father had diabetes and died of a heart attack aged 75. His father had suffered quite badly with foot problems. The patient is concerned about the possibility of having to inject himself with insulin.

Actor's Instructions

You are a 43 year old lorry driver. The reason you are visiting the practice today is to have a consultation find out the results of some routine blood tests. You are unaware that the tests have shown that you have Type-2-Diabetes.

Five years ago you were diagnosed with high blood pressure and high cholesterol and you take amlodipine 5mg/day and atorvastatin 40mg/ON.

You are aware that you are overweight at the moment and have struggled with dieting as you are unsure of where to start. Your work involves long drives and you often stop for fried food at service stations en-route. You would be willing to get advice from a dietician. You rarely have time to exercise but do enjoy playing football with your work colleagues. You have smoked 20 cigarettes/day for 20 years and drink around 8 units of alcohol/week

You are very anxious about the diagnosis of T2DM as your father who died of a heart attack at the age of 75 also had the condition. He suffered badly with foot problems. You hate the idea of having to inject yourself with insulin as you have a severe needle phobia. You know that blood sugar control is very important with diabetes but you are not sure why.

Only volunteer information regarding your concerns if you are directly asked by the candidate.

Explanation; Type 2 Diabetes

Task	Achieved	Not Achieved
Introduces self		
Confirms patient details (name, age, occupation)		
Gains consent for consultation		
Starts consultation with open question		
Takes a brief focussed history of prior events		
Asks about cardiovascular risk factors		
Gives a warning shot		
Informs patient of diagnosis		
Check's patient's understanding of condition		
Asks about patients ideas, concerns and expectations		
Explains the condition		
Explains the complications of the condition (e.g. ESRF, visual impairment, cardiovascular disease, amputation etc.)		
Explains the management of the condition (e.g. lifestyle, medications, insulin, smoking cessation etc.)		
Explains the prognosis of the condition (e.g. chronic but manageable)		
Signposts follow up and help available (e.g. diabetic nurse, patient groups, information leaflet)		
Ends consultation appropriately with summary.		
Gives patient adequate opportunities to ask questions and ensures patients' understanding of condition		
Elicits and addresses patient's concerns		
Demonstrates empathy and active listening.		
Clear structure to explanation, using jargon-free terms.		
Examiner's Global Mark	/5	
Actor / Helper's Global Mark	/5	
Total Station Mark	/30	

Learning Points

- It is important to signpost patients to additional sources of support and information such as patient support groups, information leaflets, specialist nurses and reputable websites. Especially when diagnosing patients with a chronic condition.

- In this case it is important to establish the patient's other cardiovascular risk factors as their management forms an important part of holistic care of the diabetic patient.

- It can be useful to "safety-net" patients, so they know in which circumstances to consult further medical attention.

Explaining a Procedure (Gastroscopy)

Candidate's Instructions

Patricia is a 52-year old lady attending outpatient's gastroenterology clinic for troublesome, persistent reflux. She is scheduled for a gastroscopy in two weeks' time.

You are the gastroenterology foundation doctor and your consultant has asked you to explain the procedure to the patient. You are not required to consent Patricia for the procedure, or discuss the risks associated with the procedure.

Examiner's Instructions

This is a communication station. The candidate has been asked to explain a gastroscopy procedure to a patient. They are not expected to consent the patient. Please assess their communication skills.

Patricia is a 52-year old lady attending outpatient's gastroenterology clinic for troublesome and persistent reflux. She is scheduled for a gastroscopy in two weeks' time. The patient is concerned that she may have cancer. She has not had a gastroscopy before, and is concerned about having the procedure and is adamant that she wants sedation. She is planning to drive to her son's graduation on the day of the procedure.

Actor's Instructions

You are Patricia, are a 52-year old lady. You are attending a gastroenterology outpatient appointment at the hospital as you have had a 6-month history of troublesome acid reflux. You have tried over-the-counter medications, and are taking omeprazole and ranitidine from your GP, but these have not fully alleviated your symptoms. You have lost 5lb weight over the last six months. After doing some research online, you are very worried you might have cancer.

You recently received a letter in the post with an appointment for a gastroscopy to look at your food-pipe and stomach. You have never had a gastroscopy in the past, and are anxious about what it entails and whether it will be a painful procedure. You are adamant that you want sedation for the procedure.

Other than this, you have no medical conditions or known allergies.

After the procedure, you are planning to drive across the country in preparation for your son's graduation the following morning.

Explaining a Procedure: Gastroscopy

Task:	Achieved	Not Achieved
Introduces self and explains purpose of encounter.		
Confirms patient details (name, age, occupation).		
Check patient's existing knowledge of procedure.		
Provides brief summary of procedure, reason for doing it, and approximate length of procedure.		
Takes a brief drug history to check for drugs which may increase risk of bleeding, and checks patient allergies.		
Explains the need to fast 6 hours prior to procedure and ensures patient is able to do so.		
Explains that the back of the throat will be numbed with a local anaesthetic spray, and patient may be given sedation via a cannula.		
States position: left lateral, and mouthguard worn to prevent biting of scope		
Explains: breathing will not be affected, and heart rate/O2 saturations/blood pressure may be monitored throughout.		
Explains that the patient will be asked to swallow the scope, which will then be gently advanced down food pipe to visualize structures.		
Explains that biopsies may be taken if doctor feels it is necessary, and that this will be painless.		
Provides information on post-procedure care (eating and drinking, period of monitoring/ recovery)		
Advises patient not to drive/operate machinery 24 hours post-procedure, and for someone to collect patient post-procedure.		
Inform of when/where results available and follow up		
Advise to seek medical help if becomes unwell after procedure (e.g. fever, bleeding, significant pain).		
Ends consultation appropriately with summary.		
Gives patient adequate opportunities to ask questions and ensures patients' understanding of the procedure.		
Elicits and addresses patient's concerns regarding cancer and discomfort of procedure.		

Demonstrates empathy and active listening.		
Clear structure to explanation, using jargon-free terms.		
Examiner's Global Mark	/5	
Actor / Helper's Global Mark	/5	
Total Station Mark	/30	

Learning Points

- Ensure that you elicit patient concerns and expectations early on, so you have plenty of time to address them during the consultation.

- A systematic structure is key to ensuring you provide a clear, logical explanation. Think about explaining what happens before, during and after a procedure in order to structure this station

- Familiarise yourself with common procedures that you may expected to explain, and think about how you may structure your explanation. Don't be afraid to admit that you don't know the minutiae but always offer to find out and get back to them.

Capacity

Candidate's instructions

You are the foundation year doctor on the Acute Medical unit. One of the nurses calls you to see a patient who is threatening to self-discharge. The 78 year-old patient has a background of mild cognitive impairment. They were admitted yesterday and are being treated with IV antibiotics for a UTI. The nurse asks you to speak to the patient as she is worried they haven't completed their treatment and they might not have capacity to self discharge. When you reach the patient, they have packed their bag and are sitting on the bed ready to go. They are still wearing their hospital gown and slippers and have a cannula in situ.

Examiner's Instructions

This is a communication station. The candidate has been asked to speak to a patient who wants to self-discharge. They should assess the capacity of the patient as it is in doubt. Please assess their communication skills.

The patient is a 78 years-old and was admitted yesterday. They are being treated with IV antibiotics for UTI. They have a background of mild cognitive impairment. The nurse is concerned that the patient hasn't completed their treatment and may not have capacity to self- discharge.

Actor's instructions

You are a 72-year old who is in hospital for treatment. You know you are being treated for an infection but you are unsure what exactly it is. You also know that you are in a Spanish hospital but are unsure why this is the case. The doctors have been giving you antibiotics through your cannula. You have decided that you need to go home because you need to mow the lawn and because you don't like the patient in the bed next to you, who is noisy and snores at night time. You also have a hunch that they have stolen some money from you and this morning you couldn't find your shoes and you think this other patient has something to do with it.

You can't see any point in staying in hospital, you don't feel unwell and you think the doctors are too young to know what they are doing anyway. You are not able to say what may happen to you if you do not complete the appropriate course of treatment. You have packed your bags and are waiting by your bed for a taxi.

You live on your own in a first, floor flat. You have a neighbour who helps with your shopping and a nephew who visits regularly, but no package of care.

One of those young doctors has come over to talk to you. You hope he's called a taxi for you. You are getting frustrated that you seem to have been waiting for a while, he's probably another one that doesn't understand how important it is for you to get home.

If the candidate displays the appropriate non verbal and communication skills you become less agitated and compliant with their questions, and will agree to remain in hospital for further treatment.

Capacity

Task:	Achieved	Not Achieved
Introduces self		
Correctly identifies patient		
Asks the patient an open question e.g. How are you?		
Explains purpose of discussion e.g. I've come to talk to you about you wanting to go home.		
Checks patient orientation (person/place/time)		
Clarifies why the patient wants to go home		
Asks the patient if they understand why they are in hospital		
Explains to patient importance of treatment for UTI		
Asks the patient if they understand why it might be a problem for them to go home		
Assesses if the patient can understand the information relevant to the decision		
Assesses if the patient can retain the information for long enough to make a decision		
Assesses if patient can weigh up pros and cons of decision		
Asks about social history		
Establishes patient is confused – e.g. wanting to mow the lawn but living in a first floor flat		
Clarifies how the patient would intend to get home (e.g. recognises patient is still in hospital gown and slippers with cannula)		
Identifies patient's concerns e.g. money has been stolen		
Reassures the patient		
Negotiates a plan with the patient, and closes		
Demonstrates empathy and active listening		
Demonstrates appropriate use of body language		
Examiner's global mark	/5	
Actor/Helper's global mark	/5	
Total station mark	/30	

Learning points

There is a 2-stage test of capacity.

Step One:
- The patient MUST have an impairment or disturbance of brain function.
  In this case the patient has delirium, on a background of cognitive impairment, secondary to a UTI

Step Two:
The patient has an impairment or disturbance in brain function. To be deemed to have capacity to make an individual decision they must be able meet the following four criteria:

- Understand the information relevant to the decision
- Retain the information for long enough to make a decision
- Weigh up the pros and cons of the decision
- Communicate their decision (e.g. verbally, in writing, sign language)

If they cannot meet one or more of the above criteria, they are deemed to not have capacity to make the decision.
In this case the patient was unable to weigh up the pros and cons of the decision

- Measuring capacity is decision specific: just because a patient may not be deemed to have capacity to make one decision, it doesn't mean they automatically won't have capacity to make other decisions. Capacity must be assessed for each decision individually. In the case of our patient their ability to make decisions is likely to improve as the infection clears.

- When assessing capacity every effort should be made to maximise that person's capacity such as choosing a time of day when they are alert, explaining information in a way in which they can understand, making sure they are using any sensory aids such as hearing aids or glasses.

Dealing with a complaint

Candidate's instructions

An elderly patient had a fall on the ward overnight. This was not witnessed by the nursing staff and he was found by a healthcare assistant sat on the floor. He appears to have sustained no injuries. This morning his family phoned the ward to check on his progress and were shocked to hear that he had fallen. They are very upset and demanding to speak to a doctor on the ward. They would like an explanation as to why this happened and what will be done next.

You are the junior doctor on the ward. The nursing staff have approached you and asked if you could speak with the family. Please explore the relative's concerns and offer a plan of action.

Examiner's Instructions

This is a communication station. The candidate has been asked to speak to a relative who is upset that their father has fallen whilst an inpatient. Please assess their communication skills.

The patient has had an unwitnessed fall. He was found by a healthcare assistant sat on the floor, and does not appear to have sustained any injuries. His family only found out he had fallen when they phoned the ward to check on his progress this morning. The family are upset and would like an explanation as to why this has happened and what will be done next.

Actor's Instructions

Your father is currently an inpatient being treated for a chest infection. You phoned the ward this morning to ask for an update and were told by the nursing staff that he had fallen overnight. You were concerned whether he had hit his head or fallen from a height. Unfortunately the nursing staff were unable to give you details as the fall was not witnessed by staff. He was found by a healthcare assistant sitting on the floor. They tell you he appeared to have no injuries.

You cannot understand how your father has fallen. Each day when you have visited him there has been a staff member in the bay. You are concerned that overnight the staff have 'not been paying attention' and 'care more about reading magazines'. You are particularly concerned that your father may have hit his head. You want reassurance that he has not sustained a head injury and if this cannot be offered you want to know how this will be investigated.

Your mother sustained a hip fracture following a fall in hospital the previous year. You saw how long it took for your mother to regain her confidence following this. You are concerned that your father has sustained a hip fracture and again would like this investigated. You have previously made a complaint using the Patient Advice and Liaison Service (PALS) and would like to pursue this route again.

As the doctor addresses your concerns your anger subsides. Once they explain that your father's injuries will be investigated appropriately and the cause of fall will be explored you feel relieved. You would still like to go to PALS to make a formal complaint. This is your right.

Dealing with a Complaint

Task:	Achieved	Not Achieved
Introduces self		
Confirms patient details (name, age, occupation)		
Clarifies who they are speaking to and relationship to patient and gains consent to take collateral history		
Establishes relative's understanding of events		
Explains what happened		
Makes a sincere apology		
Establish relative's concerns		
Acknowledges relative's concerns		
Reassures relative that the patient will be thoroughly reviewed and checked for injuries		
Explains that this matter will be taken seriously		
Explains that an incident report will be completed		
Explains how incident will be investigated		
Offers to escalate to senior member of medical team or nursing team		
Acknowledges relative's right to contact PALs		
Signposts how they can contact PALs		
Checks relative is happy with explanation		
Summarises next steps and closes		
Remains impartial and does not apportion blame		
Is transparent and does not embellish facts		
Demonstrates empathy and active listening.		
Demonstrates appropriate use of body language		
Examiner's global mark	/5	
Actor/Helper's global mark	/5	
Total station mark	/30	

Learning Points

- Offer an apology early on in the consultation. Remember that an apology is not an admission of guilt.

- Showing empathy, respect and listening to the relative's concerns are often more important than the content of the conversation.

- The complaint does not need to be resolved immediately. Do not try to embellish the facts. Acknowledge the unknowns and explain how the matter will be taken forward. It is sensible to arrange a follow up appointment and escalate to senior members of staff.

Duty of Candour

Candidate's Instructions

You are a foundation year doctor working on a general medical ward. Cara is a 72-year-old woman who presented with a five day history of worsening shortness of breath and productive cough of green sputum. She has been admitted to the ward for treatment for a Community Acquired Pneumonia.

Unfortunately Cara has been administered a dose of IV Co-Amoxiclav despite a documented penicillin allergy and went on to develop anaphylaxis. She received all the appropriate emergency medical management and is now stable and being monitored on HDU.

You have been asked by the nursing staff to speak with Cara's family, explaining the medication error and eliciting any concerns that they may have.

Examiner's Instructions

This is a communication station. The candidate has been asked to speak to the family of a patient who has been a victim of a serious medication error. Please assess their communication skills.

The patient is Cara, a 72-year-old woman known to have a penicillin allergy. She was prescribed and administered an intravenous dose of Co-amoxiclav earlier today, to which she developed an anaphylactic reaction. She has been managed appropriately and is now stable on HDU.

Actor's Instructions

You are the daughter of Cara, a 72-year-old girl, with known allergy to penicillin. She has been suffering with a cough, occasionally bringing up green phlegm and shortness of breath for the past five days and was admitted for treatment for community acquired pneumonia.

You were called by a member of the nursing staff to come into hospital to discuss Cara's treatment with the doctor.

You are met by the doctor in a quiet room, with a nurse present. You are informed that earlier today, Cara was given an intravenous dose of Co-amoxiclav to which she had an anaphylactic reaction.

You are furious that your mother has been put through this. You cannot understand how the mistake was made when you had clearly stated that she was allergic to penicillin on admission.

You are adamant to know the name of the doctor who prescribed the medication as well as the nurse who gave the medication. You would like to speak with them and you are considering pressing charges against them for harming your mother. You would like to know how this issue will be dealt with and how it will be prevented in the future.

You settle with reassurance that, whilst this unacceptable mistake has been made, Cara is stable and being closely monitored on HDU. You would like to know whether you can see your mother on HDU.

Duty of Candour

Task:	Achieved	Not Achieved
Introduces self		
Confirms patient details (name, age, occupation)		
Clarifies who they are speaking to and relationship to patient and gains consent to take collateral history		
Establishes relative's understanding of events		
Explains what happened		
Makes a sincere apology		
Establish relative's concerns		
Acknowledges relative's concerns		
Reassures relative that the patient is stable and being monitored in HDU		
Explains that this matter will be taken seriously		
Explains that an incident report will be completed		
Explains how incident will be investigated		
Offers to escalate to senior member of medical team or nursing team		
Acknowledges relative's right to contact PALs		
Signposts how they can contact PALs		
Checks relative is happy with explanation		
Summarises next steps and closes		
Remains impartial and does not apportion blame		
Is transparent and does not embellish facts		
Demonstrates empathy and active listening.		
Demonstrates appropriate use of body language		
Examiner's global mark	/5	
Actor/Helper's global mark	/5	
Total station mark	/30	

Learning points

- Duty of Candour is a legal duty of healthcare trusts to inform and offer remedy (e.g. apology) to patients when a mistake is made or significant harm is done during provision of a healthcare service

- Ensure detailed documentation of candid discussions is carried out including time and date of discussion, persons present, summary of the discussion and agreed next steps.

- Reassure patients and their relatives that the matter will be thoroughly investigated, and that they will be kept informed on the course and outcome of this investigation.

21604258R00152

Printed in Great Britain
by Amazon